Mastering the Transition to College

Mastering the Transition to College

The Ultimate Guidebook for Parents of Teens With ADHD

MICHAEL C. MEINZER, PhD

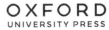

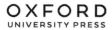

Oxford University Press is a department of the University of Oxford.
It furthers the University's objective of excellence in research, scholarship,
and education by publishing worldwide. Oxford is a registered trade mark of
Oxford University Press in the UK and in certain other countries.

Published in the United States of America by Oxford University Press
198 Madison Avenue, New York, NY 10016, United States of America.

© Oxford University Press 2025

All rights reserved. No part of this publication may be reproduced, stored in a retrieval system, transmitted, used for text and data mining, or used for training artificial intelligence, in any form or by any means, without the prior permission in writing of Oxford University Press, or as expressly permitted by law, by license or under terms agreed with the appropriate reprographics rights organization. Inquiries concerning reproduction outside the scope of the above should be sent to the Rights Department, Oxford University Press, at the address above.

You must not circulate this work in any other form
and you must impose this same condition on any acquirer

CIP data is on file at the Library of Congress

ISBN 9780197762288

DOI: 10.1093/oso/9780197762288.001.0001

Printed by Marquis Book Printing, Canada

The manufacturer's authorized representative in the EU for product safety is
Oxford University Press España S.A., Parque Empresarial San Fernando de Henares,
Avenida de Castilla, 2 – 28830 Madrid (www.oup.es/en).

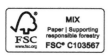

To my partner, family, and friends—thank you for all your love and support. To the many emerging adults and their families that I've worked with over the past decade—thank you for sharing your strengths, difficulties, and stories.

CONTENTS

Foreword ix
Acknowledgments xi
About the Author xii
Abbreviations xiii

PART I Introduction and Overview

1 Structure of This Guide 3

2 Communication Is Key 11

3 The ABCs of ADHD 21

4 Goal-Setting 29

PART II Organizational Skills, Time Management, and Planning

5 If It's Not on the Calendar, It Doesn't Exist 37

6 Homework 101: Effective Task Completion 48

7 How to Take Notes, Read, and Study Like a Pro 60

PART III Preparing the Application and Selecting the Right School

8 Selecting the Right School 69

9 Submitting the Application 81

PART IV Getting to Know Your Teen's Campus and Classes

10 Hiding in Plain Sight: Campus Resources 91

11 Piecing Together the Class Schedule 100

12 Academic Accommodations: What Are They Good For? 109

PART V Mental Health

13 Initiating or Maintaining Mental Health Care 119

14 Dealing with Depression 127

15 Addressing Anxiety 136

16 The Importance of a Good Night's Sleep 144

17 Alcohol Use 151

PART VI Ongoing Discussions

18 When and How to Revisit Content 161

Bibliography 164
Index 167

FOREWORD

Sending your child off to college is no doubt a stressful experience for many parents, and may feel nothing short of terrifying for parents of youth with ADHD. You may be wondering:

- Will they be able to wake up on their own and take care of themselves?
- Will they be able to meet the academic rigor of college courses?
- What if they cannot get along with their roommate?
- What if they do not keep up with their schoolwork?
- What if they don't make any friends? Or what if they make the wrong type of friends?
- What if they party too much?
- What if they fail a class?
- How will I know if they are struggling?

These concerns are normal, especially if your child with ADHD has struggled academically or socially in the past.

Many of you have played a very large role in supporting your child with ADHD through school thus far. This has obviously worked, or your child would not be thinking about college right now! You may have arranged for them to receive academic accommodations, and have coordinated care with their mental health providers, teachers, medication prescribers, tutors, and coaches for years. You may be helping them in some way with their homework and checking their grades and assignment completion online, to make sure they are staying on track. You may be picking up their medications and reminding them to take their medication each morning.

For most youth, college is a major transition period when they are living independently, away from their parents, for the very first time. Daily activities like waking up for class, eating healthy meals three times per day, going to class, getting schoolwork done, communicating with health providers and taking medications, exercising, socializing, and getting to bed at a reasonable time are entirely up to them to self-manage. As you know, ADHD is characterized by difficulty with self-management, planning, organization, and for some, impulsivity—often making this transition to independence a bit (or a lot) more challenging.

Being a parent of a teen or young adult with ADHD is also not easy. On the one hand, they want their independence and do not want you, their parents, telling them what to do. At the same time, it is so very difficult for parents—who only want their child to be happy and successful—to imagine them functioning independently. You may fear that left to their own devices they will encounter difficulty, or even fail. This is natural! It is very tempting to want to step in to make sure that they do not experience all-too-familiar ADHD-related academic and social problems.

This book is designed to help you prepare your teen for this transition *before it happens* by equipping you (and your teen) with the knowledge and strategies you can use to gradually build skills that will help your teen be successful in college and beyond. This begins with carefully considering the type of college environment that is the best fit for your child, understanding what supports are available there, and learning ways to communicate with your child in a manner that they may perceive as collaborative and supportive, rather than overbearing and directive.

I have worked with Dr. Meinzer for over a decade on research and clinical endeavors intended to help individuals with ADHD navigate developmental transitions (like the transition to college) and lead their very best lives. He has a wealth of expertise and a keen understanding of teens/young adults with ADHD that shines through in every aspect of this book. I am confident that this book can help you and your teen succeed at this exciting (yet challenging) time in their lives.

That said, it is important to accept that even when you do everything in your power to set your teen with ADHD up for success in college, there will undoubtedly be bumps in the road. This is a normal part of growing up! Framing these bumps as teaching moments and opportunities for growth will help you, as parents, to weather this big transition.

—Andrea Chronis-Tuscano

ACKNOWLEDGMENTS

As I reflect on this book, I realize there are multiple people whose contributions made this work possible. I want to express my heartfelt gratitude to Andrea Chronis-Tuscano, my mentor and friend. Your unwavering support and belief in me early in my career have been invaluable. Our shared passion for preparing students with ADHD for college led to the founding of our university ADHD clinics and also served as the inspiration for this guide for parents. Thank you for lending your thoughts to the foreword of this book.

I am also immensely grateful to Nicole Zolli for her artistic talents and clinical skills. You transformed my rough ideas into the eye-catching and informative worksheets included in each chapter. Your work has added tremendous value to this book.

I would like to acknowledge my colleagues at the University of Illinois Chicago (UIC) and particularly my department head, Jamie Roitman. Your support and encouragement have enabled me to continue serving young adults with ADHD through research studies, clinical work, and published works such as this book.

Lastly, I extend my deepest thanks to all the graduate and undergraduate students who have trained in the Young Adult and Adolescent ADHD Services Lab at UIC. Your tireless efforts have been instrumental in shaping the SUCCEEDS ADHD Clinic into the in-demand service that it is today. Your hard work and enthusiasm have been a constant source of inspiration.

ABOUT THE AUTHOR

Michael Meinzer is a licensed clinical psychologist and an associate professor in the Department of Psychology at the University of Illinois, Chicago. He is the cofounder of the SUCCEEDS ADHD Clinic at the University of Maryland, College Park and the founder and director of the SUCCEEDS ADHD Clinic at the University of Illinois, Chicago. These programs have served countless emerging adults with ADHD and their caregivers. Dr. Meinzer's research focuses on the risks associated with ADHD and developing and implementing tailored interventions to increase positive outcomes among adolescents and emerging adults with ADHD. He provides in-person and virtual trainings for clinicians and parents to address ADHD during the transition to college and maintains a private practice to stay active in treating adolescents and young adults with ADHD.

ABBREVIATIONS

ABCT	Association of Behavioral and Cognitive Therapies
ACT	American College Testing
ACT	acceptance and commitment therapy
ADD	attention-deficit disorder
ADHD	attention-deficit/hyperactivity disorder
ADHD-C	attention-deficit/hyperactivity disorder (combined presentation)
ADHD-HI	attention-deficit/hyperactivity disorder (hyperactive/impulsive presentation)
ADHD-IA	attention-deficit/hyperactivity disorder (inattentive presentation)
APA	American Psychiatric Association
APA	American Psychological Association
BAC	blood alcohol content
CBT	cognitive-behavioral therapy
CHADD	children and adults with ADHD
FERPA	Family Educational Rights and Privacy Act
GPA	grade point average
IEP	Individualized Education Plan
IT	information technology
LD	learning disability
LGBTQ	lesbian, gay, bisexual, transgender, queer
MI	motivational interviewing
NIH	National Institutes of Health
NIMH	National Institute of Mental Health
NHLBI	National Heart, Lung, and Blood Institute
OST	organizational skills training
OTMP	organization, time management, and planning
TA	teaching assistant
SAT	Standardized Achievement Test
STEM	science, technology, engineering, math

PART I

Introduction and Overview

1
Structure of This Guide

Chapter Outline

- Teaching Basic Adult Tasks
- Writing Style and Terminology
- What's to Come
- Post-Chapter Activities

If you're reading this, first and foremost, congratulations! You're nearing your teen's transition from high school to college. This is an exciting time for both parents and teens but may also be accompanied by worries about academics, communication, friendships, and juggling all of life's responsibilities. My hope is that this guidebook will help you and your teen conquer your fears and provide you with a framework for facing any difficulties head-on, having important discussions, and putting plans into place.

This guidebook is designed to prepare you to have a series of conversations with your teen as they transition from high school to college. Each chapter will focus on either an area that is important in preparing to enter college (e.g., setting goals, choosing the right school, crafting the class schedule), a common struggle for college students with ADHD (e.g., time management, organization, sleep), or a resource to be aware of while your teen is at college (e.g., academic accommodations, mental health services). Each chapter will provide an overview of the topic for parents and end with a post-chapter activity. These activities might involve discussing the topic, reviewing an infographic, or completing a worksheet together with your teen. Following the activity, your teen should take a picture of the completed ones to store on their phone or computer.

Rather than arranging chapters chronologically (i.e., from high school or pre-college through college), the book is organized into six broad topic areas. The reason for this decision is that many families will opt to have these discussions at different times depending on what is most pressing. For some families, this book will be purchased early in the process when deciding upon what colleges to apply to or preparing application materials is the priority. For other families this book will be purchased during a time when organizational concerns may be the most pressing area to address (whether teens be in high school or college). You know your family best and should approach the book in the order that you see fit.

Regarding the timeline, this guidebook is designed to initiate these discussions in the spring of your teen's junior year of high school. Beginning these discussions early with your teen will allow you more time to prepare for your teen's shift from high school to college. A sample timeline is included at the end of this chapter to serve as a recommendation for when it might be best to approach the different topics in this book. However, I also want to emphasize that if these time periods have already passed, don't worry! This timeline is not set in stone; it's just a suggestion. Content can be discussed at any time (even if your teen has already transitioned to college).

Speaking of timelines, your teen may choose to forgo entering college right away and to adhere to a less traditional timeline (e.g., taking a gap year before beginning college). If your family agrees that a gap year will serve your teen best, it's important that you and your teen develop a set of goals to make their gap year productive. These goals may consist of improving their organizational skills (with or without a professional), learning basic life skills, or working part-time or full-time to assume more responsibility (and earn money toward college). Working through the chapters of this guidebook with your teen will help to provide structure during a gap year and build a strong foundation for when they eventually enroll in college.

It is important to note that the pace of these conversations may vary from family to family. Some parents and teens may accomplish a post-chapter goal in just one conversation. Other families may need to discuss these topics in multiple conversations over days or weeks. Similarly, one chapter's activities may require multiple conversations whereas another chapter's might be able to be covered in one discussion. Further, it may be helpful to revisit these conversations once your teen has started college or during times when difficulties arise during their time at college (described in the last chapter of the book).

There may also be content that you choose not to cover with your teen. There may be topics that you do not feel comfortable discussing with your teen, like alcohol use. Though there is a strong rationale for the inclusion of each subject (as is described in each chapter), it is okay if you choose to bypass any section. It's your decision.

It is also important to consider which parents or guardians will take on the role of discussing the content with a teen with ADHD. As ADHD is highly heritable, many parents of adolescents with ADHD may struggle with executive functioning difficulties or ADHD symptoms of their own. Parents with ADHD may have a better working relationship with their child as they have a personal understanding of the executive functioning difficulties that occur in the context of ADHD. However, other parents with ADHD may be struggling with organizational skills or stress to a degree that they do not have the bandwidth to be able to offer support in these areas. Parental ADHD aside, adolescents may have different relationships with their caregivers. They may feel more comfortable discussing certain topics with one parent over another. The decision about which caregiver addresses which parts of this guidebook is important in determining how to best help with the transition to college.

Before you begin these conversations, it's also important to think about *how* you are going to approach these conversations. In the following chapter, an overview will be provided about motivational interviewing. This conversation style is suggested for parents in initiating discussions with teens in the post-chapter activities, as it may be helpful in guiding your teen toward change without having it feel like a lecture.

TEACHING BASIC ADULT TASKS

Growing up, teens assume a wide range of responsibilities. Some teens are in charge of cooking their own meals, doing their own laundry, or cleaning their bedroom or the house. On the other hand, some teens are not familiar with completing these tasks. If your teen plans to live independently, it can be helpful to teach them basic household skills before they go. Show your teen how to do a load of wash, and what to dry and what not to dry in a dryer. Hand over responsibility for their own laundry before they leave for college so as to ensure they can complete these tasks on their own when they leave home. If your teen is living off-campus (and has access to a kitchen), you should introduce your teen to a few basic meals that they can make. Though this guidebook does not have a specific chapter designated to teaching basic adult tasks (or what may be familiarly referred to as "adulting"), it is important to consider providing this instruction so that your teen can focus on academics and other life changes when shifting to college without having to worry about how to complete these tasks.

WRITING STYLE AND TERMINOLOGY

I want to provide a brief explanation for some of the stylistic choices I made in writing this book. This guidebook was written to be as conversational as possible for parents of teens with ADHD. My hope is this book will read as though I'm speaking to you directly and that this conversational style will translate to the discussions you have with your teen. When referring to your teen, I've chosen to use "they/them" as a gender-neutral, singular pronoun to be as inclusive as possible. You will also notice the term "college" used throughout the guidebook. In the United States, "college" and "university" are often used interchangeably to describe postsecondary institutions. However, outside of the United States, "college" often refers to vocational schools. In this book, I've chosen to use "college" and "university" interchangeably. Lastly, the application process for applying to postsecondary education in the United States differs from other countries (e.g., college entrance exams, and number of schools that students apply to). Though this guidebook has been written for a wide audience, there may be some aspects that are not applicable if your family is located outside of the United States.

WHAT'S TO COME

This guidebook is broken down into six parts. The remainder of Part I includes a review of ADHD (e.g., causes, symptoms, treatments), a recommended communication strategy for approaching these conversations with teens (i.e., motivational interviewing), and setting goals with teens for their transition to college (across a variety of life areas). In Part II, "Organizational Skills, Time Management, and Planning," chapters focus on helping teens implement a calendar system, learning strategies for breaking down and completing homework and day-to-day tasks, and how your teen should approach reading, studying, and taking notes in college (and as they finish high school). Part III, "Preparing the Application and Selecting the Right School," walks you through selecting schools to apply to and preparing application materials. In Part IV, "Getting to Know Your Teen's Campus and Classes," the focus will be discussing academic accommodations, campus resources (e.g., office hours, tutoring, mental and physical health care), and working with academic advisors to devise an optimal course schedule. Part V, "Mental Health," discusses a range of topics that tend to impact college students with ADHD. This includes depression, anxiety, sleep difficulties, learning disabilities, and alcohol use. Further, this section outlines the various options to address ADHD and other mental health difficulties through therapy or medication. In Part VI, "Ongoing Discussions," the guidebook will describe when and how to revisit content after the transition to college. Though designed to be comprehensive, nevertheless, this book may not be exhaustive in terms of discussions or to-do's. There may be other topics or considerations that need to be discussed if your teen has other co-occurring medical or mental health conditions, difficulties to navigate, or unique considerations. However, the following chapters are designed to be as thorough as possible and to help set you and your teen onto the road to success during their transition to college.

POST-CHAPTER ACTIVITIES

The best way to prepare for the transition to college and tackle all the associated tasks is to have an organized game plan. It's suggested that you review the included "Suggested Timeline for Success" to have an overview of the topics to cover in this book. You will also find a "Preparing for College Checklist" below. This thorough list may not be completely exhaustive, but it will provide you with the main to-do's in getting your teen prepared for the transition. Familiarize yourself with this checklist so that you can adequately plan for when to tackle each of these tasks. Finally, it is recommended that you and your teen create a digital folder where your teen stores completed worksheets. Your teen should take pictures or scan the completed worksheets in this book and store them on their phone or on their computer. This will make it easy for your teen to reference the worksheets throughout college while you maintain the copy of the book.

Structure of This Guide

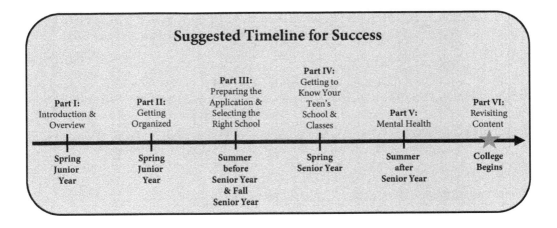

Preparing for College Checklist

Readings and Post-Chapter Activities:

- ☐ Read Chapter 1: "Structure of This Guide"
  - ☐ Review "Suggested Timeline" with your teen

- ☐ Read Chapter 2: "Communication Is Key"
  - ☐ Complete "Communication Skills Practice Quiz"

- ☐ Read Chapter 3: "The ABCs of ADHD"
  - ☐ Review ADHD Infographic with your teen
  - ☐ Complete "My ADHD Reflections: Challenges and Strengths" worksheet with your teen

- ☐ Read Chapter 4: "Goal-Setting"
  - ☐ Complete "Creating College Goals" worksheet with your teen

- ☐ Read Chapter 5: "If It's Not on the Calendar, It Doesn't Exist"
  - ☐ Complete "Organizational Skills Discussion" worksheet with your teen

- ☐ Read Chapter 6: "Homework 101: Effective Task Completion"
  - ☐ Complete "Task Completion Skills for ADHD" worksheet with your teen
  - ☐ Complete "Importance vs. Urgency Matrix" worksheet with your teen

- ☐ Read Chapter 7: "How to Take Notes, Read, and Study like a Pro"
  - ☐ Complete "Study Strategies for ADHD" worksheet with your teen
  - ☐ Complete "Reading Strategies for ADHD" worksheet with your teen

- ☐ Read Chapter 8: "Selecting the Right School"
  - ☐ Complete "Application Budget" and "College Budget" worksheets with your teen
  - ☐ Complete "Choosing a College" worksheet with your teen
  - ☐ Enter potential schools into the "School Data Table" with your teen

- ☐ Read Chapter 9: "Submitting the Application"
  - ☐ Complete "Application Checklist" with your teen
  - ☐ Have your teen record their reach, target, and safety schools on "Selected Schools" list

- ☐ Read Chapter 10: "Hiding in Plain Sight: Campus Resources"
  - ☐ Complete "Online Scavenger Hunt" with your teen

- ☐ Read Chapter 11: "Piecing Together the Class Schedule"
  - ☐ Complete "Class Schedule Builder" with your teen

- ☐ Read Chapter 12: "Academic Accommodations: What Are They Good For?"
  - ☐ Complete "Accommodations" worksheet with your teen

- ☐ Read Chapter 13: "Initiating or Maintaining Mental Health Care"
  - ☐ Complete "Mental Health Care" worksheet

- ☐ Read Chapter 14: "Dealing with Depression"
  - ☐ Complete "Coping With Depression" worksheets with your teen

- ☐ Read Chapter 15: "Addressing Anxiety"
  - ☐ Complete "Coping With Anxiety" worksheets with your teen

- ☐ Read Chapter 16: "The Importance of a Good Night's Sleep"
  - ☐ Review "Sleep Quality" worksheet

- ☐ Read Chapter 17: "Alcohol Use"
  - ☐ Review the "Alcohol Fact Sheet" with your teen
  - ☐ Decide upon and implement either the "Zero-Tolerance for Alcohol Use" or the "Protective Behavioral Strategies" worksheet

- ☐ Read Chapter 18: "When and How to Revisit Content"
  - ☐ Complete "Communication Plan" worksheet with your teen

Tasks List for Pre-College:

Application:
- ☐ Take standardized tests (ACT or SAT)
- ☐ Write college application essays
- ☐ Secure letter of recommendation writers
- ☐ Develop list of schools applying to
- ☐ Submit college applications
- ☐ Submit applications for scholarships and financial aid
- ☐ Confirm college choice in admissions portal

Mental Health:
- ☐ Talk to physician, pediatrician, or psychiatrist about continued care while teen is in college
- ☐ Talk to psychologist or mental health provider about continued care while teen is in college
- ☐ Find new professionals (if need be)

Academics:
- ☐ Sign-up for orientation
- ☐ Register for classes
- ☐ Register for academic accommodations
- ☐ Buy class textbooks and necessary school supplies

- ☐ Decide on organizational system
    - ☐ Purchase planner or calendar if physical copy is decided upon
    - ☐ Set up apps if digital platform is decided upon
- ☐ Put class schedule into calendar
- ☐ Purchase computer (if need be)

Room and Board (if applicable):

- ☐ Enroll in campus housing
- ☐ Determine meal plan
- ☐ Purchase and pack:
    - ☐ Bedding
    - ☐ Shower caddy
    - ☐ Laundry essentials (basket, detergent)
- ☐ Purchase and pack:
    - ☐ Toiletries
    - ☐ Cleaning supplies
- ☐ Decide on whether you would like to buy or rent a mini-fridge/microwave
- ☐ Determine where prescription medication will be securely stored in dorm room

2

Communication Is Key

Chapter Outline

- Collaboration Is Critically Important
- Bringing It Back to Goals
- Reflecting What You Hear
- Using Open-Ended Questions
- Staying Positive, Avoiding the Negative
- Decisional Balance
- Rolling with Resistance
- Example Vignettes
- Post-Chapter Activities

One of the most effective ways to build motivation for change is through a therapeutic technique called motivational interviewing. Motivational interviewing is used by therapists to help patients explore and resolve their ambivalence toward change, such as reasons for and against change or getting started with change. Therapists spend a considerable amount of time learning this technique, so it is unreasonable to assume that it can be taught briefly in this book. However, in this chapter I will provide a few tips (grounded in motivational interviewing) that might be helpful when talking about the topics in this book with your teen.

COLLABORATION IS CRITICALLY IMPORTANT

The conversations in this book are designed to be a team effort. In other words, it's critical to make sure that you, as the parent, do not take on an authoritative role. It's important that these discussions not seem to be directed by you but that it's truly a collaboration with your teen. For instance, rather than dictating when and what you'll be talking about, you should allow your teen the opportunity to collaborate on what topic to tackle next and to jointly decide on a convenient time to have the conversation. If your teen perceives this as a conversation with an equal voice rather than a lecture where they will be talked at, it will be far more effective. As a parent, I'm sure you've come to realize that your teen is much more likely to complete a task if it's their idea rather than if they've been told to do so. Therefore, rather than saying "We need to talk about study strategies so that you can do well on your tests," it might be more effective to ask your teen, "Why do you think it's important we talk about study strategies?" or "Why do you think this is a conversation that's recommended in this book?"

BRINGING IT BACK TO GOALS

Chapter 4, "Goal-Setting," is designed to initiate conversations about your teen's goals for their time in college. Your teen may indicate that their goals are to do well in classes, to get involved on campus, or to make new friends. Tying the purpose of the conversations in this guidebook back to your teen's goals might help to lessen their resistance. For example, if your teen is resisting a discussion on organizational strategies, you might be able to connect it to their goals for college by asking: "How do you think organizational strategies could help you do better in your classes?" or "How might having organizational strategies free up time to get involved on campus or to spend time with your friends?" This may also be true for identifying things that are not in line with their goals. For instance, if your teen indicates they wish to stop taking medications when they begin college, you might be able to connect this to their goal of doing well in classes by saying: "In what way is stopping your medication in line or not in line with you doing well in classes?" These kinds of questions and prompts will be provided in the upcoming chapters.

REFLECTING WHAT YOU HEAR

When we are having a conversation with someone, it feels good to be acknowledged. We like feeling like we've been heard! The same should be true when discussing the upcoming topics with your teen. You can use simple reflections in which you are quite literally repeating back what your teen has stated. Feeling like they've been heard may help with advancing conversations. Here's an example:

> TEEN: Putting test dates on my calendar could be helpful because then I won't have to remember it and I'll get reminders.
>
> PARENT: Your calendar could send you alerts about test dates, and it's one less thing you have to remember.
>
> TEEN: Yeah, I feel like there will be a lot of things to have to do in college, so getting reminders on my phone would be good.
>
> You can also use more elaborate reflections in which you summarize and put into your own words what you understood from your teen. You can also use a question following a reflection to keep advancing the conversation. For example:
>
> TEEN: It's going to be annoying to have to put all the test dates in my calendar. It's going to take forever! But I guess that it will make me worry less that I'm forgetting something.
>
> PARENT: So on the one hand it could take some time to put them all in your calendar, but in the long run it could be helpful so that you get reminders and don't have to worry that you're forgetting something. What other things might you want to put in your calendar?
>
> Reflections are used for more than just acknowledging what's been stated and advancing the conversation. They are also useful in that when teens hear their words

reflected back to them, they might temper their initial thoughts. Let's use the same calendar example:

TEEN: Calendars have never worked. It takes forever to put in important dates, and I don't ever go back and look at what I've put in. So what's the point?

PARENT: What I'm hearing is that there is absolutely no calendar that would work, so using a calendar would be in no way helpful.

TEEN: Well I didn't mean that. I guess the reminders part could be kind of useful.

PARENT: So the reminders might be worth using a calendar app for.

Using reflections may feel uncomfortable at first and takes practice. In each chapter you'll be given some sample prompts and reflections that you may use in the context of each conversation.

USING OPEN-ENDED QUESTIONS

Another way to advance conversations is through using open-ended questions. An easy way to describe an open-ended question is that it is a question that cannot be answered with a yes/no response. Questions that are answered with a yes/no response are closed questions. Here are a few examples of each:

Closed Questions:

Did you start writing your college application essays?
Have you asked Mrs. Arthur and Mr. Ryan to write you a letter of recommendation?
Did you look at the course catalog for your fall semester?

Open-Ended Questions:

Where are you at in terms of your college essays?
Who have you talked to so far about your letters of recommendation?
What courses looked interesting in the course catalog?

Open-ended questions open the door for teens to provide more information. Therefore, it's helpful to try and use more open-ended questions as opposed to closed-ended ones.

STAYING POSITIVE, AVOIDING THE NEGATIVE

Throughout these conversations, it's important to stay positive and avoid criticizing your teen. This may seem obvious but may be difficult at times, especially if your teen isn't willing to engage or see your perspective. Trying to take a strengths-based approach (as opposed to focusing on a teen's difficulties) might be the most effective route. For example, instead of saying "Are you sure you want to take morning classes? You can never get up on time," you could phrase that as "You seem to be able to concentrate best in the afternoon, so what classes might be best to take during that time?"

DECISIONAL BALANCE

Another technique that could be helpful in motivating teens to change is through providing a decisional balance. In other words, you'll present the pros and the cons to making a change or decision. Putting it simply, you could use the phrasing "on the one hand [reasons against or cons] but on the other hand [reasons for or pros]." The decisional balance is a helpful way of summarizing what you and your teen have been talking about, acknowledging that you're listening and that there are both positives and benefits, as well as negatives and challenges, to making the decision or change:

> [following conversation about using a calendar]
> On the one hand using a calendar takes time to set up and you will need to remember to update it. However, on the other hand using a calendar will help you manage your time better and will help to make sure you don't forget what assignments are due and when. So, what do you think?

ROLLING WITH RESISTANCE

Even if these conversations are collaborative, connect conversations to your teen's goals, and use reflective language, you may still be met with resistance. This is normal! In these cases, it is important not to push or fight back if your teen resists discussing a particular topic. Depending on the level of resistance you are facing, it may be better to reschedule the discussion for another time or revisit the conversation. However, it's also important to acknowledge with your teen that rescheduling doesn't mean that the conversation will not be revisited. See the examples of not rolling with resistance and rolling with resistance below, illustrated through short vignettes of discussions around registering for academic accommodations.

Not Rolling with Resistance:

> PARENT: So on the one hand, getting academic accommodations will require you to meet with the disability resource center and may not be necessary for every class. On the other hand, it could give you more time on tests when you need it.
> TEEN: I don't need them now. If I feel like they'd be helpful, I can always make an appointment later.
> PARENT: But you could end up failing a test because you don't have enough time. Doing it ahead of time will prevent those types of problems.
> TEEN: I already said I don't want to. I don't know how many times I have to say it!

Rolling with Resistance:

> PARENT: So on the one hand, getting academic accommodations will require you to meet with the disability resource center and may not be necessary for every class. On the other hand, it could give you more time on tests when you need it.

TEEN: I don't need them now. If I feel like they'd be helpful, I can always make an appointment later.

PARENT: Even though they could be helpful, you're confident you can do without them now. Maybe we should talk about them again after school starts.

TEEN: Yeah, okay. That works.

Ultimately you should encourage your teen to make these changes, but at the end of the day, it is their decision as an adult. The harder we push as parents or clinicians for teens to make a change, the more likely they are to push back. Our job is to help steer teens in the right direction—not take control of the wheel and steer for them. The following vignettes will help paint a better picture of these techniques.

EXAMPLE VIGNETTES

To further illustrate these communication strategies, two examples are provided below. In the first example, a parent does not use motivational interviewing techniques in talking with their son (Damien), in contrast to the second example, where they do use those techniques.

What Not to Do:

PARENT: Hey, Damien, sit down. It's time to talk about college.

DAMIEN (TEEN): I'm in the middle of watching something. Can we do this later?

PARENT: I said, now.

[Damien turns off the TV and begrudgingly walks over.]

PARENT: I thought today we could discuss your class schedule.

DAMIEN: Yeah, whatever.

PARENT: Did you look at what classes are required for your major?

DAMIEN: No. I said I'd do it later.

PARENT: Spaces may fill up quickly, and we both know that you can't handle early morning classes.

[Damien rolls eyes and starts texting on phone.]

PARENT: I pulled up the class registration website. Let's do it now.

DAMIEN: Why do you always need to take over? I said I'd do it later.

PARENT: Orientation is next week. This needs to be done now. So, it looks like you have three options for the biology class that you need to take fall semester. You should probably do the afternoon one.

[Damien continues texting while parent registers him for the class.]

PARENT: Okay. You need an elective. What about government or history? You've always done well in those classes in high school.

DAMIEN: I don't want to take history. It's always so boring.

PARENT: You really should take a history class. You need something that will be easier for you to bring up your grades. Do you want to do US history or European? They're both in the afternoon and fit in your schedule.

In this example, there were quite a few instances where the communication was not in line with the collaborative approach we are aiming for. Specifically, the parent takes the lead, asks closed-ended questions, and uses some critical language. The next vignette provides examples that are in harmony with optimal communication strategies.

A Prime Example:

PARENT: Damien, it's about five minutes until noon. We agreed we'd be talking about your class schedules then. Just wanted to give you a heads-up.
[Five minutes passes.]
PARENT: All right, Damien, let's get started. Join me at the table, please.
DAMIEN (TEEN): What are we doing again?
PARENT: Class registration for the fall is now open and you have an advising appointment at orientation next week. What have you thought about so far?
DAMIEN: Well, I know I'd like to major in biology, so a lot of the classes are already decided for freshmen.
PARENT: Great, so it seems like you've already done some of the groundwork. What would you want to do first? Look at the required science classes or look into your elective classes?
DAMIEN: I guess we can do the electives.
PARENT: Great, where do you think we should start?
DAMIEN: Well, the biology website said I need to take an English class.
PARENT: Okay, let's start with English. Where do we see what classes are available?
DAMIEN: The registration website, duh.
PARENT (IGNORING THE "DUH"): Okay, will you pull that up?
DAMIEN: So here are the English classes. There's one on science fiction at 9 a.m. on Mondays, Wednesdays, and Fridays. That seems cool, but I hate waking up early.
PARENT: That does seem like a class you'd enjoy, but it sounds like you don't think the timing will be ideal. Any others that look interesting to you?
DAMIEN: Not really. The noon class on Tuesday and Thursday is a better time but I don't think I'm going to like the topic. Poetry isn't really my thing.
PARENT: So, on the one hand the science fiction class would be more engaging, but you'd have to wake up earlier than you'd like. On the other hand, with the poetry class, you'd be able to sleep in, but you might find it boring. What do you think? What's more important to you? The class or the time?
DAMIEN: I mean probably the class, but I hate waking up that early.

PARENT: Yeah, getting up early has always been a bit of a struggle for you but I'm confident you can manage. At some point, would you be open to talking about some ways to help get you up in the morning?

POST-CHAPTER ACTIVITIES

To practice some of the skills grounded in motivational interviewing, complete the practice quiz below. The quiz is designed to help reinforce some of the communication skills discussed in this chapter.

Remember to mark off the completion of this chapter and the corresponding worksheets on the "Preparing for College Checklist" in Chapter 1.

Communication Skills Practice Quiz

1. **Match the teen statements to the parent reflections**

Teen Statement	Parent Reflection
a. I hate math classes.	1. Not planning things out ahead of time can lead you to being really overwhelmed with work, and that impacts a lot of areas of your life.
b. I've never needed extra time on tests before. I don't think I need them in college.	2. Balancing school and your social life will be a priority for you when you start college.
c. I get really stressed when I'm doing things right before the deadline, and that really impacts my sleep.	3. Being on your own and independent seems to be a really important part of your college decision.
d. I usually just complete the review packet to study for a test. Sometimes I use flash cards.	4. Since in high school you didn't need academic accommodations, you feel in college things will be the same.
e. I want to move out and live on campus. I'd really like to live in a new city.	5. Math classes seem to be really challenging for you.
f. I obviously want to do well in classes, but I also want to make friends and get involved in Greek life.	6. Active study strategies seem to be most helpful. If professors provide a study guide that would be ideal, though in college that might not be likely.

2. **Which of the following are open-ended questions?**
   a. Did you register for accommodations yet?
   b. What calendar system do you think would work best for you?
   c. What do you know about the symptoms of ADHD?
   d. Do you think evening classes are a good idea?
   e. Do you want to continue seeing your therapist during college?
   f. How might breaking things down help you get started on tasks?
   g. Where do you find it's easiest to get work done?
   h. One of your goals for college is getting good grades, right?

**Bonus: try revising the closed questions into open-ended ones.

3. **Below is a scenario describing a teen and parent conversation about academic accommodations. Based on the information provided, write a decisional balance statement.**

   Teen and parent are discussing using academic accommodations and whether or not they might be helpful for the teen when they begin classes. During the conversation, the teen says that the amount of paperwork to get accommodations seems tedious and that they've never had to use accommodations in high school. Teen does note that the tests and work in college are likely to be harder than in high school and they want to get good grades.

   _____

   _____

   _____

   _____

   _____

4. **True-False.** When your teen pushes back on having a conversation, the best approach is to just direct the conversation and power through.

Communication Skills Practice Quiz Answers

1. **Reflections**
   a. 5
   b. 4
   c. 1
   d. 6
   e. 3
   f. 2

2. **Open-Ended versus Closed Questions**
   - Open-ended questions: b, c, f, g
   - Closed questions: a, d, e, h
     - Changing closed to open:
       a. Did you register for accommodations yet? ➔ Where are you at in the registration process for accommodations?
       d. Do you think evening classes are a good idea? ➔ What time of day do you think you're able to pay attention best in class?
       e. Do you want to continue seeing your therapist during college? ➔ What are the benefits of continuing to see your therapist?
       h. One of your goals for college is getting good grades, right? ➔ What are your goals for your time in college?

3. **Decisional balance**
   On the one hand, filling out the paperwork for accommodations will take some time and you might not necessarily need them for all your classes, but on the other hand the tests and assignments in college are probably going to be more difficult. You also mentioned that your goal was to get good grades in college, so having them in place may be a good safety net in case you need them. What do you think?

4. **Rolling with resistance**
   FALSE: Being authoritative may backfire and have your teen push harder against the topic of conversation. It may be best to reschedule or revisit the conversation at a mutually agreed upon time. However, this does not mean your teen is off the hook. The conversation still needs to happen; it just needs to happen at a more appropriate time.

The ABCs of ADHD

Chapter Outline

- What Is ADHD?
- What Causes ADHD?
- How Does ADHD Impact College Students?
- Strengths
- What Can You Do?
- Example Vignette
- Post-Chapter Activities

Before discussing the various topics and skills that will be presented in this book, it's important to provide an overview about attention-deficit/hyperactivity disorder (ADHD) and the potential difficulties that teens with ADHD often encounter. It's possible that many teens are unfamiliar with this information. If teens are treated for ADHD in fast-paced settings, they may not have received a thorough explanation of what ADHD is or how it may affect different areas of their life. Therefore, it may be helpful to share this information with your teen or have a conversation to fill in the gaps. The post-chapter activities and infographics will help to guide you through conversations about ADHD symptoms and to identify your teen's strengths and difficulties.

WHAT IS ADHD?

ADHD (formerly known as attention-deficit disorder or ADD) is a neurodevelopmental (i.e., brain-based) disorder that generally begins to affect individuals in childhood or early adolescence and may continue to impact them into adulthood. ADHD symptoms fall into three categories: inattention, hyperactivity, and impulsivity. Which symptoms an individual experiences determines the diagnostic presentation. Individuals with the predominantly inattentive presentation (ADHD-IA) tend to have difficulties paying attention, following through with tasks or instructions, and make careless mistakes. They may experience some symptoms of hyperactivity or impulsivity, but not clinically significant levels. The second presentation is characterized by hyperactivity or impulsivity (ADHD-HI). Individuals with ADHD-HI tend to be fidgety or restless, talk too much, interrupt others, and act before they think. They may experience some symptoms of inattention, but not clinically significant levels. The last presentation is characterized by having a combination of high levels of inattention, hyperactivity, and impulsivity (ADHD-C). Symptoms of ADHD are typically present early in life, but they may not cause a person difficulty until much later (like high school or college) when demands in their life become more challenging. Many individuals with ADHD also tend to struggle with executive functioning difficulties. "Executive functioning" is a term that describes a set of mental skills that include planning, organization, attention shifting, and self-control.

WHAT CAUSES ADHD?

ADHD is a brain-based disorder. There are differences in not only the levels of certain brain chemicals among people with ADHD but also differences in how certain areas of the brain function. These brain areas are usually responsible for thinking, planning, organizing, and regulating emotions and behavior. ADHD also tends to run in families because of its genetic basis. When discussing what causes ADHD, it's equally important to discuss what doesn't cause it. ADHD is not caused by too much sugar, food additives, or allergies. Though parental support and scaffolding may decrease ADHD-related impairment, parenting behaviors do not cause ADHD.

HOW DOES ADHD IMPACT COLLEGE STUDENTS?

The following information is based on research studies where college students with ADHD and their peers without ADHD were evaluated. The results of these studies are not meant to suggest that your teen with ADHD will definitely experience these outcomes. This information is just to report possible experiences your teen may be at an increased risk for. For instance, college students with ADHD are more likely to experience various greater academic difficulties (e.g., time management) compared to their peers without ADHD. This could look like having trouble with knowing what assignments are due and planning out when and how to do them in advance of a deadline. Inside the classroom, students with ADHD may have difficulty completing tests in the same amount of time compared to their peers without ADHD.

College students with ADHD are also susceptible to difficulties outside of academics. For example, college students with ADHD are at greater risk for experiencing anxiety, depression, sleep difficulties, and alcohol-related negative consequences than their peers without ADHD. These concepts are discussed in more detail in chapters in Part V, "Mental Health." There may also be difficulties managing day-to-day tasks outside of academics. Maintaining a consistent schedule for managing daily responsibilities (like eating, cleaning, doing laundry), seeing therapists, and taking medications may also be more difficult for college students with ADHD.

These academic, mental health, and personal difficulties may stem from the shift in supports that teens were accustomed to receiving in high school. In the academic realm, there are likely many supports in high school that may have protected against negative consequences:

- Teachers checking in with students if assignments were not turned in
- Consequences for not attending class (e.g., detention, call home to parents)
- Open lines of communication between teachers and parents
- Teachers assigning smaller tasks that build to a larger assignment (e.g., being assigned sections of an essay that are turned in regularly over the course of weeks or months)

- Class schedules where teens are accounted for throughout the day
- Having time to complete homework in class or in school

As students transition to college there are natural changes in the types of supports they were once accustomed to receiving. College students may now be taking classes in large lecture halls where attendance isn't tracked, and professors may not reach out if assignments are not turned in. They may have large breaks in their schedule that require them to be productive or stay motivated to return to class later in the day. They may need to now create a game plan for completing a large assignment (e.g., project, essay) without interim due dates built in by professors. They also now need to be advocates for help from professors and teaching assistants or to receive academic accommodations.

From a social perspective, teens also likely received structure and support from being under the same roof as their parents or support from an established friend group. This may have come in various forms:

- Friends excusing ADHD symptoms that impact their relationships (e.g., interrupting, forgetting to text back or follow through)
- Friends reminding your teen to turn in assignments, follow through on tasks, or attend activities
- Parents being aware of their teen's behavior (e.g., when they are completing homework, when they are attending school)
- Parents being able to communicate more easily with both teens and their teachers
- Parents being able to assist with homework or daily living tasks

Upon entering college, teens may no longer be living with parents, making communication more difficult. Phone calls or texts may need to be planned since there is not the likelihood of natural interactions throughout the day. Parents won't be hearing from their teen's professors throughout the semester. In fact, under the Family Educational Rights and Privacy Act (FERPA), when teens enter a postsecondary institution, educational rights transfer from parents to the teens themselves. This makes it challenging for universities to share educational records or information with parents without the consent of the student. Providing support to college students may also become more difficult as parents try to balance providing the monitoring and supports students need to be successful with the independence they desire.

STRENGTHS

I want to also emphasize how your teen has unique strengths that you should be mindful of while discussing their difficulties and the skills that may help them reach their full potential in college. Throughout your teen's life they have likely been keenly aware of areas where they struggled (whether it was their own perception, based on grades received, or what they heard from teachers or family members). While knowing areas of difficulty may be helpful in determining where the introduction of skills would be helpful, it is equally important to highlight students' strengths and successes. For instance, parents should acknowledge their teen's perseverance and ability to overcome their ADHD-related difficulties. As you work through this book with your teen it is important to reinforce the areas where they excel as well as the fact that they have successfully navigated the path to college.

WHAT CAN YOU DO?

Despite these challenges and the changes that are bound to occur during the transition to college, there are a wide array of resources that are available to your teen, skills that they can learn, and ways that you may appropriately support your teen during this developmental transition. This guidebook will discuss ways you can advocate for your teen in terms of university resources on university campuses (e.g., academic accommodations, tutoring, advising that takes into account their ADHD-related strengths and difficulties; see Chapters 10–12). This guidebook will also describe what skills-based (e.g., organizational skills training, cognitive-behavioral therapy, academic coaching) and pharmacological (e.g., stimulant medication) interventions you and your teen may elect to pursue through mental health providers in the community (see Chapter 13). Further, this book will also introduce skills that you may use to directly support your teen as they leave high school and enter college.

EXAMPLE VIGNETTE

The following vignette is included to provide you with an example as to how you could introduce the infographic to your teen. In this example you will read about how the parent and teen discuss causes of ADHD, symptoms of ADHD, the ways symptoms of ADHD impact day-to-day functioning, and Justin's unique strengths. You'll also note that the parent in this example uses the communication skills outlined in the next chapter (e.g., open-ended questions, reflections).

> PARENT: Justin, let's take a look at this worksheet together. At the top here, it goes over the causes of ADHD. Over the years, what have you learned about the causes of ADHD?
>
> JUSTIN (TEEN): Well, to be honest, not a whole lot.
>
> PARENT: This book talks about how people with ADHD have a brain that works just a bit differently, which can cause some trouble with paying attention, following through on tasks, being organized. Those sorts of things.
>
> JUSTIN: I guess I assumed it had something to do with the brain, but I never really knew.
>
> PARENT: Yeah, and it also says here that there are many different ways that the symptoms of ADHD may present themselves. There are symptoms of inattention, symptoms of hyperactivity, and symptoms of impulsivity. People with ADHD may have a combination of these symptoms or just symptoms in one area. What types of symptoms do you feel you recognize the most?
>
> JUSTIN: I don't think I'm hyperactive or anything. At least not anymore. Maybe as a kid I had more of those hyper symptoms. I would say mostly now I just have trouble paying attention.
>
> PARENT: Okay, so these days it's less of the hyperactive and more of the attention type symptoms. It says in the book that that's pretty common; a lot of teens phase out

of the hyperactive type symptoms in their adolescent or young adult years. So how do the troubles with paying attention affect your day-to-day life?

JUSTIN: I don't think they do.

PARENT: Trouble paying attention doesn't impact you at all.

JUSTIN: Well, I guess that's not totally true. Sometimes I forget to turn stuff in and it's hard for me to pay attention in some classes.

PARENT: So even though it may not be every day, it may impact some parts of your schoolwork.

JUSTIN: Yeah, I guess so.

PARENT: Even though ADHD makes school a little harder for you, it's important we talk about your strengths too.

JUSTIN: What kind of strengths?

PARENT: Your personal strengths. Things you're good at. Things you accomplish even if having ADHD makes it more difficult.

JUSTIN: Well, I feel like I'm creative.

PARENT: You are really skilled in music and art! What else?

JUSTIN: I don't know. I guess I'm smart, I got into college.

PARENT: That's an excellent point. You are so intelligent and even though school may be challenging sometimes, you've stuck with it and persisted! Getting accepted into college is no easy feat.

JUSTIN: True. I never really thought of it that way.

PARENTS: Knowing the things that are challenging is the first step at figuring out what we should do to make sure you're successful in school. But it's also important to acknowledge all your strengths too! As we work through this book, I want us to both keep in mind both the challenges and the strengths that are unique to you.

Hopefully this sample vignette provides a helpful framework for discussing information about ADHD. Though some of the information in this chapter and in the corresponding infographic may already be familiar to your teen, for many this may be the first time that they've had a discussion about what it means to have ADHD.

POST-CHAPTER ACTIVITIES

After reading this chapter, schedule a time with your teen to review the "What Is ADHD?" infographic which illustrates the causes, symptoms, and difficulties associated with ADHD. Following this conversation, discuss the ADHD-related difficulties and strengths your teen experiences using the "My ADHD Reflections: Challenges and Strengths" worksheet. These may be related to their academics (e.g., in-class, completing assignments, reading), work (e.g., completing work, making it to shifts on time), social life (e.g., difficulty following through with commitments, trouble with following conversations). On the same worksheet, it's important for you and your teen to discuss their unique strengths (e.g., perseverance, creativity, talents).

Following these discussions, try to reinforce one strength your teen exhibits, one success your teen achieves, or one effort your teen makes in the next week. Remember to mark off the completion of this chapter and the corresponding worksheets on the "Preparing for College Checklist" (see Chapter 1). Be sure to have your teen save a picture of the completed worksheets in the designated spot on their phone or computer.

WHAT IS ADHD?

ADHD is a brain-based condition caused by...

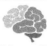

Structural differences. Key brain regions like the prefrontal cortex, basal ganglia, and cerebellum show differences in activity and structure that impact executive functions and emotion regulation.

Chemical differences. Neurotransmitters are chemical messengers in the brain. Dysregulation of these messengers in ADHD (e.g., dopamine, serotonin, norepinephrine) impairs attention, mood regulation, and reward processing.

Genetic differences. ADHD is highly heritable, as it is commonly passed down through numerous genes. This means that if someone in your family has ADHD, it's more likely that you have it too.

ADHD is NOT caused by too much sugar, food additives, allergies, or a specific parenting style.

The **Diagnostic and Statistical Manual of Mental Disorders (DSM-5)** lists the following criteria for ADHD:

ADHD Inattentive Symptoms
1. Makes careless mistakes.
2. Struggles to sustain attention.
3. Doesn't listen when spoken to.
4. Doesn't follow through on instructions or tasks.
5. Has trouble organizing tasks.
6. Avoids sustained mental effort.
7. Often loses necessary things.
8. Easily distracted by surroundings.
9. Frequently forgetful in daily activities.

ADHD Hyperactive/Impulsive Symptoms
1. Frequently fidgets and squirms.
2. Leaves seat when remaining seated is expected.
3. Runs or climbs excessively.
4. Can't play quietly.
5. Always "on the go."
6. Talks excessively.
7. Often blurts out answers.
8. Can't wait their turn.
9. Often interrupts or intrudes on others.

Someone can be diagnosed with ADHD-Inattentive type (ADHD-IA), ADHD-Hyperactive/Impulsive type (ADHD-HAI), or ADHD-Combined type (ADHD-C). Symptoms emerge before age 12, are present across different settings (e.g., school, home, work), and negatively impact social, academic, and/or occupational activities.

These symptoms can lead to...

- trouble with daily responsibilities
- academic difficulties
- organization and time management difficulties
- mental health and sleep issues

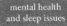

My ADHD Reflections: Challenges and Strengths

Reflecting on your ADHD-related challenges and strengths is a great way to understand yourself! Figuring out what situations or tasks are tough for you and why, as well as embracing the strengths you undoubtedly have, will help you overcome obstacles in the future. Use the columns in this worksheet to write out and reflect on these parts of yourself.

ADHD-Related Challenges	Personal Strengths
Reflecting on challenges related to your ADHD means looking at tough situations honestly, then planning steps to manage them better next time—every outcome is a step toward your growth.	Recognize what you're naturally good at, use these skills to boost your confidence, and don't shy away from showing others your unique abilities—they're powerful assets in every challenge.

1. _____
2. _____
3. _____
4. _____
5. _____
6. _____
7. _____
8. _____
9. _____
10. _____

1. _____
2. _____
3. _____
4. _____
5. _____
6. _____
7. _____
8. _____
9. _____
10. _____

4

Goal-Setting

Chapter Overview

- Types of Goals
- Example Vignettes
- Post-Chapter Activities

To master the transition to college, it's important to first define what a successful transition is! A successful college career can be defined in many ways. One way students can determine their college success is to assess whether they achieve or attempt to achieve their goals. These goals may be short-term (e.g., a daily or weekly goal), mid-term (e.g., a semester or yearly goal), or long-term (e.g., by the end of college). Success can and should be defined across many life areas. A student's life can be broken into numerous domains: academics, work, social life, daily responsibilities, and self-care. It would be unreasonable of anyone to judge success by evaluating only one of these life areas. Therefore, it's important to determine what goals your teen has across *multiple* areas to have a more comprehensive view of success.

TYPES OF GOALS

The first—and perhaps most obvious—way to define success in college is via academics. Academic success may be defined as getting certain grades, obtaining a certain GPA, turning in a certain percentage of homework on time, attending class, and so on. It's important to have academic goals at each of the previously mentioned stages: short-term, mid-term, and long-term. Short-term goals could consist of submitting 80% of assignments on time each week (without needing an extension), studying 20 minutes per day in a particular subject, or attending all classes each week. Mid-term goals could consist of achieving a B or better in each class, attending office hours once per course in a semester, completing prerequisite classes to transfer into a new major, or registering for academic accommodations. Long-term goals could consist of completing a study abroad experience, finishing college, graduating with honors, or securing a job before finishing school.

Students should also have goals within the social domain (e.g., maintaining and forming relationships). In the short term, this might be calling or texting friends from high school and family members each week to stay in touch, attending club meetings or rehearsals once a week, or eating one meal with a new college friend each day. Mid-term goals might consist of joining a new club by the end of the semester, rushing a fraternity or sorority, or increasing their network of friends. Long-term goals might be pursuing a romantic relationship or fostering relationships with professors who will write a strong letter of recommendation for graduate school or job applications.

During college, students may also hold a part-time or full-time job, and if so, they should have goals related to this area of their life too. These goals may consist of arriving to work (on time) for every shift in the short term, working toward a promotion or moving into a different department in the mid-term, or securing an internship that will help them to obtain a job post-graduation in the long term.

Students should also be sure to determine goals related to their own self-care (i.e., doing things that will help your teen take care of their physical or mental health). In the short term, this could consist of taking medication daily, exercising several times per week, or attending therapy appointments. Mid-term goals might be scheduling an evaluation for medication for ADHD, finding a mental health therapist, or attending annual or semiannual doctor's appointments. Long-term goals might include training for an event (e.g., a marathon or 10k) or learning how to cook healthy meals and meal-prep.

Students may also want to set goals for taking care of their household responsibilities (i.e., chores or responsibilities with their living situation). In the short term, this could consist of putting clothes in their hamper each day, doing laundry once a week, or cleaning their room once a month. In the mid-term and long term, goals could include finding a new living situation (e.g., different dorm, different roommate) or living off-campus in their own apartment.

You may be wondering why it's so important to outline these goals. The reason is that throughout this book you should tie your discussions about skills and behaviors to these specific goals. The more your teen relays the purpose of these discussions back to what they want to accomplish, the more likely they are to buy into this process and put in the work for a successful transition. For example, your teen may question the utility of discussing one of (or all) the chapters in this book. My hope is that you will respond in a way that ties the conversation back to their goals. Here are a few examples of how you might be able to do so (while using some of the communication skills discussed in Chapter 2).

EXAMPLE VIGNETTES

Example 1:

> REBEKAH (TEEN): Why are we even doing this? Why do I have to talk about class schedules with you?
> PARENT: How do you think your class schedule will impact your college goals?
> REBEKAH: I don't know.
> PARENT: Well, a few months ago we talked about what your goals were for college. What do you remember?
> REBEKAH: I guess one of them was that I wanted to do well in my classes.
> PARENT: Exactly. You said you wanted to get a B or better in your classes. How do you think your class schedule might impact your ability to do well in your courses?
> REBEKAH: Well, if I take too many hard classes at once, I might not be able to keep up.

Example 2:

> CALEB (TEEN): I just don't get the point of planning out when I'm going to do my work. If it needs to get done, it will get done.
> PARENT: Mind if I share some thoughts, Caleb?

CALEB: I guess not.

PARENT: One of the reasons the book suggests planning out when you're going to do work is that planning may help you be more efficient. Why might it be helpful to be more efficient?

CALEB: You get work done quicker.

PARENT: Right! And what's the benefit of getting work done quicker?

CALEB: You have more free time.

PARENT: Yes, exactly. With more free time you'd be able to pursue more of your nonacademic goals like pledging a fraternity or joining the ski team.

Example 3:

TRISH (TEEN): I don't understand why we're talking about sleep. I'm not even at college yet.

PARENT: To you, it seems early to address this. Any thoughts as to why sleep is included? How has sleep affected you in high school?

TRISH: I mean when I don't sleep well it's hard for me to pay attention.

PARENT: So not having enough sleep could make it hard for you to perform well in class and ultimately could affect your GPA. I remember you saying your goal was to try and keep your grade about a 3.0.

TRISH: Yeah.

PARENT: How might not getting enough sleep affect your goal of being on the crew team?

TRISH: The practices are super early in the morning.

PARENT: So not going to bed early means it could be hard for you to wake up in the mornings or you might be tired during the day. So, you might miss practice and could end up having trouble with your schoolwork.

Example 4:

PARENT: It seems like you're hesitant to register for academic accommodations.

REUBEN (TEEN): I don't think I need them.

PARENT: Let's think about them in the context of your goals you decided on. Remind me, what was your academic goal?

REUBEN: I think I said I want to make sure I am above a 3.0 so I can transfer into the business school.

PARENT: Okay, so scoring high on exams and getting your homework in on time are key factors that will impact your GPA.

REUBEN: True.

PARENT: Do you think that accommodations could help your GPA or even be a safety net if you experience any difficulties with an assignment or on exams?

Tying these conversations back to your teen's specific goals may help to motivate them to put in the time and effort of having these conversations and engaging in the post-chapter activities.

POST-CHAPTER ACTIVITIES

To set the stage for a successful transition, a goal-setting worksheet is included at the end of this chapter. Complete the "Creating College Goals" handout with your teen to reveal your teen's short-term, mid-term, and long-term goals across their different life areas. This will likely take one or more conversations. You don't want to overwhelm your teen with too much content all at once. Therefore, you may want to start with one life area (e.g., academics) and discuss the short-term, mid-term, and long-term goals. On a separate occasion, you could talk with your teen about a different life area (e.g., social life) and complete the goals for that topic. You and your teen know best in terms of how many areas to address in one sitting but be mindful of trying to cover too much ground in one discussion.

Remember to mark off the completion of this chapter and the corresponding worksheets on the "Preparing for College Checklist" (see Chapter 1). Be sure to have your teen save a picture of the completed worksheets in the designated spot on their phone or computer.

Creating College Goals

Goal-setting is a crucial skill for the transition to college. It helps young adults clarify what success means to them, focus their energy and attention on tangible outcomes, and make it easier to prioritize tasks and projects. Use this worksheet to first create long-term goals and then to create short-term goals.

The Big Picture

Creating long-term semester and yearly goals provides structure and continuity to your entire college journey. In the time frames below, record 1–3 goals.

By the *end of college*, I would like to have accomplished the following goals:

NOTE: This worksheet is designed around a two-semester system across five years. If your college uses a different system (e.g., a quarter system) or you plan to graduate within a different time frame (e.g., four years), please adjust this worksheet accordingly.

YEAR 1 GOALS	By the end of my **first year**, I would like to have...	
	During my 1st semester, I want to...	During my 2nd semester, I want to...
YEAR 2 GOALS	By the end of my **second** year, I would like to have...	
	During my 3rd semester, I want to...	During my 4th semester, I want to...
YEAR 3 GOALS	By the end of my **third** year, I would like to have...	
	During my 5th semester, I want to...	During my 6th semester, I want to...
YEAR 4 GOALS	By the end of my **fourth** year, I would like to have...	
	During my 7th semester, I want to...	During my 8th semester, I want to...

YEAR 5 GOALS	By the end of my **fifth** year, I would like to have...	
	During my 9th semester, I want to...	During my 10th semester, I want to...

Weekly and Daily Goals

Creating weekly and daily goals helps you manage tasks efficiently and stay motivated to meet both short-term and long-term goals. In the time frames below, record 1–3 goals.

	WEEKLY GOALS By the end of this week, I would like to have...
WEEK OF:	
	DAILY GOALS By the end of the day, I would like to have...
Monday	
Tuesday	
Wednesday	
Thursday	
Friday	
Saturday	
Sunday	

PART II

Organizational Skills, Time Management, and Planning

5
If It's Not on the Calendar, It Doesn't Exist

Chapter Outline

- Pros and Cons of Organizational Systems
- Types of Organizational Systems
- What Goes Into an Organizational System?
- When to Initiate and Maintain Organizational Systems
- Troubleshooting
- Example Vignette
- Post-Chapter Activities

Though it may be obvious to some, developing and maintaining an organization system is crucial for college students, especially for those with ADHD. Unfortunately, this is an area of difficulty for many college students with ADHD. As mentioned in Chapter 3, many emerging adults with ADHD struggle with executive functioning. Organization is one area under the umbrella of executive functioning. Helping your teen develop an organization system will help to lay the foundation of their college success. For the purposes of this chapter, "organizational systems" refers to things such as planners, calendars, and to-do lists. Beginning this discussion during high school (e.g., the spring of their junior year; see Chapter 1), may be particularly helpful so that your teen has time to practice these skills before entering college. However, if this timeline has already passed, that's okay too. Introducing these skills at any point will certainly be helpful, though the earlier the better so that your teen has opportunity to practice and implement a system. This will also allow you and your teen time to find a mental health professional (see Chapter 13) should circumstances warrant it.

PROS AND CONS OF ORGANIZATIONAL SYSTEMS

With any important decision, it's important to acknowledge both its pros and cons. It may seem like there aren't any cons to developing an organizational system, but it is important to discuss this area with your teen. To begin the discussion of developing an organizational system, it may be helpful to engage in a decisional balance exercise (see Chapter 2). Specifically, you could begin by asking your teen what they dislike about using an organizational system (e.g., planner, calendar, to-do list) or challenges they may encounter. One common concern that students typically describe is the effort and time that comes with starting and maintaining an organizational system. This is a fair argument. Using a planner, calendar, or to-do list *does* require diligence. First, students need to think about what type of organizational system they want to use. Then, it takes time for them to write down or input an assignment on their calendar or to-do list. It may seem like a daunting task, especially at the beginning of the semester when there are class times, assignment due dates, and exam dates for many courses as well as other nonacademic events (e.g., group meeting times, doctor's appointments).

In addition to inputting dates and times into a calendar or planner, it may also be difficult for them to check and maintain it. Putting in due dates and important times into a calendar is a meaningless task if it's not referred to. Ensuring that dates and times are being monitored and that new dates and times of events are being entered as they come about could be time-consuming. Your teen may also describe feeling overwhelmed when they see a to-do list or a calendar full of time blocks. It is important to acknowledge these concerns and validate your teen before discussing the pros.

After discussing the downsides to calendar use, it's time to discuss the positives. As you can imagine, there are a lot of upsides to using an organizational system. First, it allows students with ADHD to not have to hold all of this information in their head. It is almost impossible to remember all the class times, due dates, and exams for each of their courses on top of nonacademic events. Having a place to store this information will allow students to focus their energy on other things without worrying they're forgetting about something. An electronic calendar system also provides alerts or reminders for upcoming due dates or appointment times. These methods may help students in not missing class or forgetting to complete assignments. To-do lists also help to itemize what assignments need to be completed. Often, they are even built into online calendar system platforms (more to come on these in the next section). Being more in tune with important dates may also lead to improvements in academic performance.

Initiating the discussion about both the pros and cons for organizational systems will help to potentially motivate your teen to adopt some sort of planner, calendar, or to-do list. The worksheet at the end of this chapter should be used as a guide for this conversation. Detailed directions for completing this worksheet are provided in the "Post-Chapter Activities" section. After developing the pro/con list, your teen may or may not be ready to implement all the necessary pieces of an organizational system. It is important to meet your teen where they are at (Chapter 2) and slowly build upon their organizational system. It may not be as thorough as you'd like, but it may be a start. You can always revisit their organizational system at a later date or discuss calendars over the course of several conversations. The next section outlines some examples of organizational systems that your teen may be willing to adopt. If all fails, it could be helpful to work with a mental health professional to help encourage your teen to improve organizational skills.

TYPES OF ORGANIZATIONAL SYSTEMS

In the spirit of collaboration, it is important to not force an organizational system on your teen but to work with them to help them decide on one they feel will be feasible for them to adopt. The following section describes some of the various types of organizational systems. It is important to try and elicit types of organizational systems from your teen. After they contribute to the list, you can fill in any missing ones from this chapter. After creating the list, it will be helpful to talk about the pros and cons of adopting each of the organizational systems. Ultimately, this discussion should end with your teen selecting one or more of these systems.

Paper Calendars and Planners

Paper calendars and planners may be seen as old-school to some but helpful to others. Some teens like to carry around a planner with them and go through the physical act of writing an assignment down and crossing it off. This may be especially true for students who may not be particularly tech-savvy. Though any organizational system is better than none, there are some downsides to using a paper planner or calendar. First, it requires that students carry this planner to every class. If they don't have it with them, they would have to remember to add it to their planner later—which somewhat defeats the purpose of a planner in the first place. It also requires that they write appointments many times over (e.g., having to write down class times each week for an entire 16-week semester). Planners often have space in which students can write down tasks that need to be completed for the week. This format may be helpful, so that students will see what they need to do and then schedule a time to complete it in their planner all at the same time.

As a substitute or in conjunction to using a physical planner, some students opt to adopt a desk or wall calendar. On the desk or wall calendar, ideally they put important dates (e.g., exams, appointments) and use a planner to outline when they are going to do a task each day. However, it would likely only be helpful when students are at home. A desk calendar will not be able to alert them as to where they should be or what they should be doing when they are away from it. Another option for students is to use a notebook to create a to-do list and use a planner or calendar to keep track of important dates. The downside with this option is that students will have to remember to carry around multiple things with them to all their classes, and they will likely not have these items with them in social settings.

Electronic Calendars and To-Do Lists

Electronic organizing platforms (e.g., Apple Calendar, Google Calendar, Trello) have many features that maximize efficiency. These platforms most often have web-based platforms (to use on one's computer) as well as app-based platforms (to use on one's phone). This allows for someone to enter appointments, tasks, and due dates while at home working on schoolwork or on the go. In this digital age, students are likely carrying their phone with them at most, if not at all, times. This allows students to update their calendar or to-do list at all times. Further, it will sync with any web-based platform that they are able to access on their computer. An additional benefit of using an electronic platform is that they have the capability for recurring appointments to be added (e.g., every Tuesday and Thursday from 12:00–1:00 for an entire semester). Recurring appointments only require students to enter a class once and have it carried over across the semester. These app-based programs will remind students of upcoming events or due dates (e.g., your teen could receive an alert 15 minutes before class time). Students can also color-code based on the types of activities (e.g., red for classes, green for work hours, blue for extracurricular activities). Importantly, many of these apps can be used free of charge.

Electronic to-do lists may help to complement calendar use. Apps like Google Tasks, Apple Reminders, Notes, and Trello will list what tasks need to be completed. Having a to-do list will help to ensure that your teen is not missing assignments by visually presenting all necessary tasks that need to be completed (and by what date and time). Students can prioritize what needs to be done by having it higher on the to-do list. Additionally, to-do lists can be linked with calendars (e.g., Google Tasks can appear as a sidebar on Google Calendar; to-do lists and calendars appear within the same app in Trello; Apple Reminders can sync with Apple Calendar). Students can add tasks to their task list at any time, assuming they are carrying their phone.

Less Optimal Options

As stated above, any organization system is better than nothing. However, the following options may be less optimal than the ones listed above. Using sticky notes (or Post-its) as reminders may be helpful in some settings (e.g., having a sticky note reminder on your teen's desk to remember to check their email), but it may not be helpful to have many sticky notes placed all over a desk or dorm room that contain various tasks or reminders. Sticky notes are also designed to stay in one place. Though it may be that your teen is reminded of a task when they are at home due to the placement of the notes, it is unlikely they will be reminded from sticky notes when they are not home. Sticky notes may also become unstuck from places and thus no longer serve their purpose as reminders.

Bullet journals are another popular though often less ideal option. Bullet journals are notebooks in which individuals draw in their own organizational framework. For example, someone starts with a blank page in a notebook and draws out different sections (to-do lists, a goal tracker, space to reflect). In theory, this is a fantastic approach to combine a to-do list with a space for your teen to detail their goals or reflections. However, often individuals spend hours drawing out these sections and decorating their pages rather than actually completing the tasks that they need to do. In other words, bullet journals may be used as a procrastination tactic—something that is extra salient for students with ADHD.

Occasionally, teens will want to use multiple calendars and planners (e.g., one planner for academic tasks and one planner for nonacademic tasks; one calendar for academic appointments and one calendar for nonacademic appointments). Though this means they would have all the necessary information marked down, they would also have to check multiple places to make sure they have completed all tasks or do not have any obligations. Therefore, it's preferred to have everything in one spot so that there is only one place to have to remember to check.

WHAT GOES INTO AN ORGANIZATIONAL SYSTEM?

Once you and your teen have discussed the various types of organizational systems, it's important to decide what elements need to be included. The best way in which to initiate this discussion is by asking your teen what they think should be included on a calendar. After your teen lists the elements that they think belong, you should ask to share any remaining items from the section below.

Classes, Appointments, and Obligations

First and foremost, getting class times on the calendar is essential. This has several advantages. Having it on the calendar will help to ensure that classes aren't missed. Electronic calendars provide reminders for classes times (e.g., a phone vibrating 15 minutes before class begins). Students should also enter the location of classes within the calendar event.

In addition to class times, it may be helpful to enter appointments (e.g., meetings with an advisor, professor office hours, work hours). This not only helps to decrease the likelihood that class or appointments are missed but also helps to visually lay out what time your teen has free to engage in extracurricular and recreational activities, or to complete homework.

Completing Tasks

It may also be helpful for students to schedule time to complete their work assignments. Though it could be helpful to block off general time (e.g., 3 hours) to complete homework, it is far more helpful if your teen blocks off specific time for each assignment (e.g., 1 hour to complete math problems, 1 hour to write the introduction of their paper, 1 hour to read their creative writing text). More information on breaking down tasks can be found in Chapter 6. Having the time to complete assignments as well as classes and other events on their calendar will help to visually present students with the amount of free time that they have unobligated throughout the week. Students may need assistance with estimating the amount of time it takes to complete a task early in their college career. When having this discussion, you should ask your teen to draw on previous experience in high school or in college in completing similar tasks to estimate the amount of time needed. You may also want to encourage your teen to overestimate the amount of time to allot to complete an assignment. It's always better to finish ahead of schedule than to not finish a task within the scheduled time.

Due Dates and Exams

In addition to weekly events like classes or blocking off time to complete work or engage in nonacademic activities, putting due dates on the calendar is equally important. The most efficient organizational systems include when assignments are due, when exams and quizzes are being held, and any other important course-related deadlines. This will allow students to juggle many course-related demands and map out their week ahead of a deadline. Having due dates listed decreases the likelihood of missed assignments, last-minute surprises, and the need to pull an all-nighter to complete work.

Daily Responsibilities ("Adulting")

There are likely other tasks that students will need to complete outside of academics. These activities of daily living are especially important to be mindful of if a student is living in the dorms or independently off-campus, but may also apply to students living at home. These responsibilities may consist of cleaning, doing laundry, exercising, and running errands (e.g., picking up prescription medication). Students should also consider how and when they will eat their meals and what other steps that may entail. If living at home, it may consist of merely budgeting time to eat prepared meals with family. If living in the dorms, it may consist of dedicating time to commute to a dining hall to take meals. If living independently off-campus, it may consist of planning time to grocery shop, prepare food, and eat. Planning time to complete the tasks that they may not be used to completing independently will be important in ensuring they successfully navigate all aspects of college life and independence.

WHEN TO INITIATE AND MAINTAIN ORGANIZATIONAL SYSTEMS

In addition to discussing the "what," it's also important to discuss the "when" of organizational system initiation and upkeep. This topic should start with an open-ended question asking your teen when they think the best time would be to enter all the information into their organizational system. It also may be helpful at this point to remind your teen that this process could be time-consuming, but reiterate the benefits (pros) they completed on their worksheet.

Proactive Completion

The ideal time to enter class times, assignment due dates, and exam dates would be the first week of the semester. Typically, the first week of the semester tends to be slightly lighter in terms of homework responsibilities. This is an optimal time to take each course syllabus and input all important dates throughout the semester as well as all class meeting times. By entering all of their class times, due dates, and exam dates into their organizational system, students will not have to remember things or have to enter these pieces of information throughout the semester.

Reactively

Even if students input all the important and relevant information into their to-do list and calendar, other assignments, appointments, and obligations will inevitably come up throughout the semester. There are several options for keeping their organizational system up to date. Ideally, students would enter the information immediately. For instance, students could enter any appointment or additional assignment as soon as they learn about it (e.g., at the end of class). This reduces the risk that these items don't make it onto the calendar or to-do list. However, this is only feasible if students are carrying their phone or planner at the time. Students likely carry their phone at most times, which might be another reason for your teen to opt for an electronic system.

Alternatively, though somewhat less ideal, students could enter the new obligations or assignments at a designated time or times during the day. For instance, students could enter in new tasks at mealtime (e.g., lunch or dinner). Alternatively, students could reflect on all the new tasks they need to complete for the next day before bed. However, the downside to this approach is that items could be forgotten before they are entered.

TROUBLESHOOTING

When discussing your teen's new organization system, it's important to acknowledge that developing a new habit takes time and effort. Students likely need support to stay consistent. Therefore, it's important that you and your teen identify who will support them and how they will provide support. This is an important component to the overall discussion. The last portion of this conversation should be dedicated to helping your teen identify potential roadblocks as well as who can help them overcome any organizational difficulties. Support can come in different quantities and from a variety of people. Your teen may feel they need daily check-ins, weekly check-ins, or support on an as-needed basis. These check-ins may occur electronically (e.g., via text or email), in person, or via telephone. This level of support may also need to change throughout the semester. For example, during the beginning of the semester students may feel they need more frequent check-ins, as they are learning how to organize their responsibilities. However, they may want to reduce the frequency of these check-ins mid-semester or mid-year as skills are mastered. Alternatively, students may realize they need more support if they feel things are slipping throughout the semester. Therefore, it will be important for your teen to identify in your conversations how they will know if things are going well with their organization, how they will know if things are not going well and need extra support, and who they will reach out to when they need more accountability.

You and your teen should also discuss which individuals they want to rely on for support on their organizational journey. First, and perhaps most obvious, parents can often be a powerful source of support. Parents know their children better than anyone else and have a full history of their strengths and difficulties when it comes to organization. They are often the most invested in their child's success and likely have the greatest access. How to carry on this organizational support is discussed in detail in the final part of this guidebook (Chapter 18).

Some teens may be resistant to having check-ins with parents. Therefore, it's important for you and your teen to come to an agreement about the level and degree to which you will be involved in their organizational system. If there is resistance to parental support in terms of organization, your teen should identify alternative individuals who may be able to assist with encouraging consistency and troubleshooting. This could be a close friend or sibling that your teen would feel comfortable working with.

In addition to this somewhat informal support, there also may be support within your teen's college that could help with organizational skills such as the writing center, disability resource center, or other specialty clinic (see Chapter 10 for campus resources). It may be helpful for your teen to continue to build their organization skills with a mental health professional or ADHD coach. See Chapter 13 for more information on what to look for in a helping professional who has expertise in ADHD. This may be especially true if your teen has struggled with organizational skills in the past.

EXAMPLE VIGNETTE

The following vignette depicts a conversation between a parent and a teen regarding setting up an organizational system.

> PARENT: I'm hoping we can spend some time talking about organizational systems. Let's start with where things are now. How do you keep track of your homework assignments and important dates now?
>
> LORI (TEEN): Well, most of the time I just remember, or you remind me. Sometimes I have to write things in my planner if the teacher has us pull them out in class.

PARENT: Okay, so it sounds like sometimes you use your planner but most of the time you don't. What are the things you don't like about using your planner, or any organizational system for that matter?

LORI: Most teachers don't give us time in class to write things down and I have to rush out to my next class. Mr. Mobley is the only one that ends early so we can write things down.

PARENT: Time is a big factor for being able to record it all in the moment. What else is a downside to using a planner or app on your phone?

LORI: I've just never needed to use it before. It's all online or I remember.

PARENT: So, the workload in high school hasn't been hard enough to warrant needing one. How might using one be helpful in college, where the workload might be more challenging?

LORI: Like you said, I'll probably have more work and more classes I need to keep track of.

PARENT: Right, what else?

LORI: I mean you won't be around to remind me, so I have to rely on something different.

PARENT: So, on the one hand it takes time writing things down and getting the system set up but on the other hand it could be helpful for remembering all of the things you have to do. What do you think?

LORI: I'm willing to try, I guess.

PARENT: You mentioned your school planner, but I'm curious if there are other types of organizational systems or apps you've heard of.

LORI: I know Vincent uses an app on his phone a lot. He seems to like it.

PARENT: Some of your friends have had success with electronic organization systems.

LORI: Yeah, I think if I'm going to use a planner in college, it has to be on my phone.

PARENT: Seems like an easy decision then. Great! What kinds of things do you think you would want to put on your calendar?

LORI: When I have class seems important.

PARENT: I agree. That seems super important. What else?

LORI: Due dates, maybe?

PARENT: I like that idea too! What about things like when you're going to spend time on homework?

LORI: I don't know, that seems messy. I don't want to add too much.

PARENT: What do you think the pros and cons of blocking off time to do work would be?

This conversation highlights just a few pieces of the organization system discussions you'll want to have with your teen. The post-chapter activity will guide you and your teen through the various components of a potential organization system.

POST-CHAPTER ACTIVITIES

As has been discussed in prior chapters, the conversation around organization may require multiple conversations to adequately cover the material in this chapter. Working collaboratively with your teen, please complete the "Organizational Skills Discussion" worksheet. This worksheet will outline the pros and cons to using an organizational system, the types of organizational systems your teen could use, and the details of initiating and maintaining that system. If you need a refresher about possibilities, refer back to the corresponding sections of this chapter before discussing with your teen.

Remember to mark off the completion of this chapter and the corresponding worksheets on the "Preparing for College Checklist" (see Chapter 1). Be sure to have your teen save a picture of the completed worksheets in the designated spot on their phone or computer.

Organizational Skills Discussion

What are the pros and cons to using an organizational system?	
Cons:	**Pros:**
1. _____	1. _____
2. _____	2. _____
3. _____	3. _____
4. _____	4. _____
5. _____	5. _____

What are types of organizational systems?	

What type of organizational system is the best fit for you?

What should go on the calendar?	

When will things be added to the organizational system throughout the semester (e.g., in the morning, at night)?

Who will help with executing this plan?

How will I know if things are going well with organization?

How will I know when I need extra organizational help?

6

Homework 101

Effective Task Completion

Chapter Outline

- Creating the Right Environment
- Prioritizing Tasks
- Breaking Down Tasks into Specific and Manageable Pieces
- Maximizing Productivity
- Rewards
- Post-Chapter Activities

Now that you and your teen have discussed what type of organizational system may work best for them, it's important to discuss the best ways for your teen to tackle the tasks on their calendar or to-do list. This chapter will outline some tips students should use in completing homework assignments. However, the skills presented in this chapter are merely an introduction. Your teen may need to work with a professional or tutor to really hone these skills. Regardless of whether this specialized support is needed, the first step is for you and your teen to be familiar with effective ways for them to complete tasks.

CREATING THE RIGHT ENVIRONMENT

The first step to completing tasks, is finding the environment that is most conducive to working or studying. The ideal environment will likely differ from student to student and may even change based on their mood or type of work that needs to be completed. Knowing what works best for your teen will help to set them up for success.

Location

Where to complete work is an important consideration. It may be difficult to know ahead of time (i.e., before your teen arrives to college) where the optimal location will be. However, you and your teen may be able to reflect on what's been effective thus far. For some students, especially those with ADHD, being in a private space may be most conducive to getting work done. Throughout adolescence, this type of setting may have been a quiet study hall at school, the library, or a quiet room at home (e.g., study or bedroom). Less optimal places that your teen may have been getting work done throughout high school could be the lunchroom or rooms in the house where there are distractions (e.g., the television, family members talking).

In college there will be a variety of places to get work done. Each of these places may come with pros and cons. One of the most obvious places may be students' bedrooms (i.e., either at home if they are commuting or in the dorm if they are living on campus). Though it may seem to be a convenient spot, there may be challenges to completing work in their dorm room or bedroom at home. First, they may have roommates (or a sibling or other family members) who could serve as a distraction. Even if roommates are not disturbing them, their presence may make it more difficult for students with ADHD to complete work. Students likely also have electronic distractions in their room (e.g., computer, television, video games), which are likely far more entertaining than completing homework. If students are tired, they may be tempted to lay down in bed or attempt to complete work in bed. This could inadvertently lead to an unplanned nap or downstream sleep difficulties (see Chapter 16). Therefore, even though it may be less convenient to leave their room to get work done, it may be the best option if they are easily distracted. Encouraging your teen to find a place outside of their room to complete work may help to increase their productivity (more on this in the coming paragraphs).

Alternatively, if working in their dorm room (or their bedroom at home) should be the only option or your teen is adamant on working in their room, there are some things your teen could consider to make their room as conducive as possible for completing work. Students may want to consider using noise-canceling headphones or ear plugs to block out any distracting noise. They may want to consider shutting down electronics (e.g., computers, video games) or moving them to a place outside of their work area to minimize potential distractions. Having a designated workspace in their room (i.e., a desk or table) is important to avoid the potential of doing work in their bed.

Many students find it helpful to find a place outside of their room on campus to complete work. Completing work outside of their room not only tends to increase productivity but also creates a natural boundary between home (i.e., their room where they can relax and not think about work) and school (i.e., where they take classes and complete homework). This allows their home to be a place of relaxation or enjoyment not tainted by the pressure of completing schoolwork. There are many places on campus students can select as their designated workplace. The library may be one that comes immediately to mind. University libraries typically have many floors with differing workstations. Some floors are designated quiet areas whereas others allow for talking softly between students. Some have large tables with multiple people working at them where others have private cubicles. Regardless of whether students like a completely silent space or a space where there is some background noise, the library is one place your teen might want to consider for completing work. Additionally, universities also have multiple libraries around campus (e.g., the main university library, college- or school-specific libraries). Therefore, your teen may have several options if a library is their desired workplace or they'd like a change of scenery but still work within a library.

If the library seems intimidating or too quiet, there are many other locations on campus that students can take advantage of. There may be lounges within a student's dorm building, coffee shops close by, or the student union. Throughout your teen's first semester you should encourage them to explore campus to find a space that works best for them. This may also include asking friends or upper-level students where they like to get work done.

Accountability Partners

In addition to location, it is also important to discuss with your teen if (and when) they find it helpful to complete work or study with a peer. Accountability partners can be peers, classmates, or family members who can help to keep a fellow student on track with work completion. An accountability partner may be working on the same assignment or just completing work simultaneously. The presence of an accountability partner may help with not only motivation to get started but also encouragement to persist. Accountability partners can work in person or even over a video or phone call. This idea has also been referred to as "body doubling." Communities have formed online where individuals can body-double with each other (sometimes with a membership fee to join) through an organized platform.

On the other hand, there are likely peers that might serve as a distraction for your teen getting work finished. If your teen is more likely to talk with a friend or get sidetracked than get work done, they may not be a great choice for an accountability partner. Therefore, helping your teen identify the people (or the traits of people) that may make a good accountability partner may be helpful in increasing their productivity.

It may be too early for your teen to know who at school would be good in this role. They may be an entering freshman and enrolling in a school where they don't know anyone yet. In that case, it may be helpful to revisit this section when they have started to form a social network. In the meantime, you might help them identify people currently in their life that could serve as an accountability partner during their high school years or remotely (e.g., via video call) when they begin college.

Other Factors That Impact Productivity

There are a few other miscellaneous environmental factors that may affect your teen's ability to get work done. A student's energy level is a clear element for productivity. Therefore, it's important for students to make sure they have eaten or have snacks with them throughout their work session. Being hungry or thirsty may serve as a distraction so making sure they have these basic needs met is critical. Similarly, if students take prescription medications for ADHD (e.g., stimulants), it's important that they've taken their medication prior to beginning a challenging task. Your teen should build a strong internal environment for beginning a study session.

Another consideration is whether music or ambient noise would be helpful for your teen. Some students find music to be helpful while others may find it distracting. The type of music also might play a role; lyrics could be distracting for some, so instrumental music or ambient noise (e.g., white noise, rain sounds) may be what a student opts for. For others, any type of noise is distracting so ear plugs or noise-canceling headphones are necessary.

Your teen's ideal environment may also differ depending on the type of work that needs to get done. For example, writing an essay might require a different setting (e.g., quiet, at a desk, working alone) compared to completing a math assignment (e.g., working with a classmate). Therefore, it would be helpful for you to discuss these various scenarios with your teen so that they have a game plan for the different types of work that will arise throughout their college career. The post-chapter activity includes a guided discussion of this topic.

PRIORITIZING TASKS

In college, your teen will have to juggle many responsibilities. There will be homework to complete, tests to study for, and essays to write for multiple classes. Often these due dates will coincide, and your teen will have to decide what work to complete first. There are many strategies when it comes to prioritizing. It may be tempting for students to complete the easiest task first. Though this could help them get the ball rolling with starting their homework, they may be spending time on a task that is not as time-sensitive or significant to their grades. Similarly, it may be appealing to take on household chores (e.g., cleaning, doing laundry, organizing) as a way to delay getting started on a difficult academic task. Therefore, it may be helpful to work with your teen on learning how to prioritize their work. One effective way is to prioritize by how important a task is and how time-sensitive the matter is.

Importance

One of the criteria to be considered when prioritizing is the importance of each task. Importance may be defined by the weight of an assignment in one's grades. If two assignments are due at the same time, it may be in a student's best interest to focus on the assignment that carries more weight (e.g., writing an essay worth 100 points should be completed before doing an assignment worth 20 points). However, it may also be important to consider an assignment's impact in the context of a specific course. The number of points may not be the only matter worth considering. For example, a 20-point assignment may be more important if a student is in jeopardy of failing that class or on the cusp of achieving a higher grade. Those sorts of extenuating circumstances may impact a student's decision-making around significance. Though number of points may typically work as a measure of importance, there may be other factors that should be considered in making the decision about what assignment gets priority based on importance.

Time-Sensitivity

In addition to importance, time-sensitivity also needs to be considered. As with importance, it may be tempting to complete the easiest task first (even if it's not due for several days) while ignoring the difficult assignment that is due tomorrow. Therefore, teens need to consider when the deadlines for assignments are and how much time it will take to complete them. Typically, the assignment due first should be prioritized. However, as was mentioned in the discussion of importance, there may be other things to consider. For example, perhaps one assignment is due tomorrow but an essay that is not due for two days will require significantly more time. In those instances, the amount of time required could factor into the decision-making process.

Combining Importance and Time-Sensitivity

There may be some scenarios where only importance *or* urgency are at play; where two scenarios have the same level of one construct but varying levels on another construct (e.g., two assignments have the same due date but are worth different point totals; two assignments are worth the same number of points, but one is due in one day and one is due in three days). In most cases, students have to weigh importance *and* urgency. Of these scenarios, the easiest one would be when the most important thing is also due soonest (e.g., an essay worth 100 points is due tomorrow and the math assignment worth 20 points is due in several days). However, there may be instances that are more challenging (i.e., when one assignment is more important but less time-sensitive; when one assignment is more time-sensitive but less important). Therefore, it's important for your teen to ask themselves questions to determine the best place to start. When tasks are roughly equal in their importance and urgency your teen may have to make a thoughtful decision on where to start. The post-chapter activity on importance and urgency will help your teen practice this fact-finding mission so that they are more confident in the way they prioritize their assignments. For some students, this exercise may be enough in learning how to prioritize. For most, continued practice will be necessary. This may come in the form of guided discussions with you during the semester or through working with a professional (e.g., therapist, ADHD coach; see Chapter 13).

BREAKING DOWN TASKS INTO SPECIFIC AND MANAGEABLE PIECES

Once your teen has decided on the assignment to complete, it may be helpful for them to break down the assignment into smaller, more manageable tasks. With any difficult or lengthy task, it can often feel overwhelming getting started. Writing a 10-page paper from scratch or catching up on all the reading for a test (e.g., 5 chapters) can seem daunting. Further, when a task like this seems insurmountable, it may be easier to get started when there is a more achievable first step. Your teen will want to consider what the first piece of the task is and ensure that it is more easily accomplished. For example, rather than putting "write 10-page essay" on the to-do list, your teen could break this task into much smaller ones: "outline paper," "write thesis statement," "write 1 page," and so on to "write conclusion." The same should be done for tasks requiring reading and studying. Rather than blocking off time with a generic task of "studying," your teen could indicate what and how they will study: "make flash cards, complete chapter 1 homework problems, complete chapter 2 homework problems, complete practice test."

By breaking down the task into more manageable parts, it can make the process of getting started easier. It can also help your teen to feel accomplished throughout completion of that task. In other words, they can continue to cross items off the to-do list throughout the process. This mere act can help to reinforce on-task behavior and keep their momentum going with their homework. Some teens with ADHD may struggle with dividing a task into smaller pieces. In the beginning, it may be helpful for parents (or a mental health professional) to assist teens in this process to develop a more detailed task list collaboratively.

After breaking down tasks, your teen should set 1–3 reasonable goals for studying or reading during a task block. An example of this might be: (1) reading pages 75–85 in a math textbook and (2) completing math homework problems. Following the completion of this task block, your teen should reward themselves with a short break before beginning another task block. These task blocks may help the work seem more reasonable and allow for needed breaks in between completing assignments. These breaks should be timed, so that a planned 10-minute break doesn't end up turning into much longer. After the break time is over, your teen should set a new 1–3 goals for the next task block.

If your teen finds it challenging to even set a goal of one task block, they could consider using a variation of the Pomodoro method. For example, your teen could set a timer a goal to work for 20 minutes and allow themselves to take a short break (e.g., 5 minutes) afterward. Once the 20-minute work timer goes off, your teen should evaluate if they need a break or if they can persist and complete another 20-minute task block. When your teen decides to take a break after a task block, they should set a timer and resume the 20 minutes of work when the break is over. Your teen should repeat this process until their work is complete.

Some students excel in making plans to complete work but struggle with executing them. They may know what to do but become stuck when they sit down to begin the task. In these instances, having someone to hold them accountable may help immensely (see the "Accountability Partners" section above). In some instances, it may be necessary for parents to take a more active role in helping teens complete their homework. Parents may consider establishing coworking sessions with teens with ADHD to help hold them accountable for executing their plan for completing homework. If this level of parental support seems too invasive for teens, parents and teens should schedule check-ins with teens (e.g., once a day, once a week, multiple times over the weekend) to help them stay accountable with executing their plan, problem-solve any difficulties, and re-plan if necessary. These types of monitoring might be helpful when teens struggle with executing the planned tasks or meeting their work session goals.

Like prioritizing, breaking down tasks and setting reasonable goals may also be complicated for teens. Though the post-chapter activity will help your teen to practice this process, your teen may need ongoing consultation. Therefore, you and your teen may need to schedule a time each week (or each day) to identify work that needs to be completed, practice breaking homework assignments down, and schedule when those assignments or tasks will be completed. Alternatively, and perhaps more optimally, your teen could work with a mental health professional or ADHD coach to hone this skill.

MAXIMIZING PRODUCTIVITY

Now that we've covered finding an appropriate space and environment to complete learning which tasks to prioritize, and setting manageable goals, it's important to share some tips that are helpful for students in maximizing their productivity. There are likely times of the day that your teen may feel fresher. Some teens are morning people—they have the best concentration abilities when they first wake up. Others feel best in the afternoon, especially if they are prescribed stimulants and their medication has had time to reach maximal effectiveness. Some students feel most effective in the evening hours. It's important for you and your teen to discuss the times of day when they feel most and least productive. Within this context it's also important to discuss what topics typically require the most and least focus. Ideally, your teen will schedule the task that requires the most concentration during the time that they are most fresh. Though this is something you should certainly encourage and help your teen to plan out, they may need expert consultation with a mental health professional, ADHD coach, or peer mentor.

Another helpful tip is making use of time in between obligations. For instance, if students have an hour in between classes, that is an opportunity for them to finish work that can be completed in a short amount of time. For example, they could choose to answer emails, review flash cards, complete an assignment while on a break in between classes. By completing work while in "school mode," students will have more time at the end of the day to pursue extracurricular activities, relax, or socialize with friends. Making use of these times is an efficient way to complete work and have a balance between school and social life.

Similarly, it could be helpful for your teen to stay on campus or go to a study space (e.g., the library) after classes before going home. Often, when students go back home to their dorm or apartment they get comfortable, begin watching television, and get distracted. It then becomes more difficult to get back into school mode. By avoiding the temptations at home, they are likely to be more efficient.

REWARDS

Whether it's receiving a sticker for completing chores as a school-aged child or getting a yearly bonus as an adult for meeting job performance goals, rewards can be incredibly motivating. Rewards are a means of positively reinforcing productive behavior. When a child gets a sticker for completing a chore or an adult gets a bonus for meeting work goals, it's more likely that in the future those productive behaviors (e.g., getting chores done, completing work tasks) will happen again. In college, this may look like a student buying their favorite meal after homework is completed.

One way of implementing positive reinforcement is through the Premack principle. The Premack principle is based on the assumption that a more preferred or desirable activity can be used to encourage the completion of a less desirable or preferred activity. A simple example of the Premack principle is a parent telling their young child, "If you eat your vegetables, then you can have dessert." In college, this may look like students committing to finishing their homework before going to a party. Positive reinforcement and the Premack principle can be challenging for college students in that it is up to students themselves to only engage in the more preferred activity when the less preferred one is completed. However, parents should encourage college students with ADHD to apply this principle and monitor whether students are abiding by their self-imposed rules (e.g., not spending time with friends until their essay is written).

POST-CHAPTER ACTIVITIES

This chapter covered a variety of techniques for maximizing student productivity. It's unlikely that you will be able to complete all the post-chapter worksheets in one sitting. Therefore, you may want to reserve more time to cover the post-chapter activities than in chapters past. First, you and your teen should review the "Importance vs. Urgency Matrix" and complete the worksheet using examples from your teen's life. The "Task Completion Skills for ADHD" worksheet will require you and your teen to further discuss prioritizing tasks. You and your teen should discuss finding the right environment to complete work, maximizing your teen's productivity, and breaking down tasks into more easily achievable pieces.

Remember to mark off the completion of this chapter and the corresponding worksheets on the "Preparing for College Checklist" (see Chapter 1). Be sure to have your teen save a picture of the completed worksheets in the designated spot on their phone or computer.

Importance vs. Urgency Matrix

A Time Management and Decision-Making Tool

College is full of tasks that compete for your attention, which may make it difficult to know where in your workload to begin. The Importance vs. Urgency Matrix helps you categorize tasks based on their importance and urgency to prevent "ADHD paralysis" and optimize time management.

Importance refers to how *significant or impactful a task or activity is* in relation to your goals, values, and long-term objectives. Important tasks contribute directly to your personal or professional development, well-being, and overall success.

Urgency refers to how *time-sensitive a task or activity is*. Tasks with a higher level of urgency require immediate attention and action to prevent negative consequences, avoid missed opportunities, or meet deadlines. These tasks often have short-term implications and may not necessarily be aligned with your long-term goals.

Take a look at the example below. Then try this activity yourself, using the blank template provided and any school assignments or household tasks you must do this week.

	URGENT	LESS URGENT
IMPORTANT	**Do it now.** Study for my exam tomorrow Pay rent that is due tonight Emergency doctor's visit for allergic reaction	**Schedule a time to do it.** Laundry (I have about a week until this is urgent) Work on long-term project Schedule study sessions for final's week
LESS IMPORTANT	**Seek an extension on the task, or delegate it to someone else.** Attend a minor club meeting tomorrow Complete a noncritical favor tonight for a classmate	**Consider removing it from your schedule.** Watch a TV show Browse YouTube

Importance vs. Urgency Matrix
A Time Management and Decision-Making Tool

Use the template below to organize the various tasks you must complete in your life. Remember that **importance** refers to how significant or impactful a task or activity is in relation to your goals, values, and long-term objectives. Meanwhile, **urgency** refers to how time-sensitive a task or activity is.

	URGENT	LESS URGENT
IMPORTANT	Do it now.	Schedule a time to do it.
LESS IMPORTANT	Seek an extension on the task, or delegate it to someone else.	Consider removing it from your schedule.

Task Completion Skills for ADHD

Strong task-completion skills are essential to a successful college experience. Developing these skills will reduce feelings of overwhelm around work, improve your time management, reduce stress, and boost your academic performance. To begin, you might find it helpful to review the strategies below. **Consider the skills below and check the box next to 1–2 skills you will try for one week. Answer the questions marked with a star (★) to guide your thinking.**

	PRIORITIZE your tasks
☐	**Use a centralized task list** ■ Color-code or write a symbol next to 2–3 priority items
☐	**Prioritize tasks by importance and time-sensitivity** ■ *Important items* impact your goals, values, and long-term objectives ■ *Time-sensitive* items may need to be done immediately or urgently
☐	**Prioritize tasks based on what is efficient, realistic, and feasible** ■ *Efficient* processes achieve maximum productivity with minimum wasted effort ■ *Realistic* processes are practical and achievable within given constraints ■ *Feasible* processes are possible and capable of being accomplished
☐	**Review and adjust your priorities regularly** (*) **How often should you review your priorities** (e.g., once a day, during the task)? _____
☐	**Utilize the "two minutes" rule** ■ If you can do something in under two minutes, go ahead and do it right that moment!
	Choose the right ENVIRONMENT
☐	**Identify your ideal work environment** (*) **When do you work best** (e.g., morning, night)? _____ (*) **In what places do you get your best work done** (e.g., home, library, cafe)? _____ (*) **In what type of environments do you get your best work done** (e.g., quiet environments, environments with music or white noise)? _____ (*) **With whom do you get your best work done** (e.g., a studious friend, alone)? _____

	PRIORITIZE your tasks
☐	**Minimize distractions** ▪ Remove electronic distractions (such as a phone or tablet) from view ▪ Wear noise-canceling headphones
☐	**Have a designated workspace outside your bedroom** ▪ Avoid working in your bedroom, as it can be especially tempting to complete nonwork activities (e.g., sleeping, scrolling on the phone) ▪ Alternative spaces include the library, a coffee shop, or other buildings on campus
☐	**Establish routines and rituals around homework**
☐	**Choose an accountability partner** (*) Who might be a good accountability partner? _____ (*) What traits does a good accountability partner have (e.g., working on the same assignment, is generally focused on work)? _____ (*) What traits does a poor accountability partner have (e.g., prone to distraction, uninterested in work)?
	Maximize PRODUCTIVITY
☐	**Meet your basic needs**—*work with your body, not against it!* ▪ Avoid hunger by eating before work or having snacks while working ▪ Avoid thirst by drinking water before work or while working ▪ Take any medications you might need
☐	**Complete challenging tasks when you tend to feel best** (*) What time of day do you have the most focus? _____ (*) What time of day do you have the least focus? _____ (*) What type of tasks (e.g., reading, writing) **require the most effort to focus?** _____ (*) What type of tasks (e.g., drawing, math) **require the least effort to focus?** _____
☐	**"Chunk" tasks to meet your attention span** ▪ When feeling fresh, chunk steps so that they are longer or more complex ▪ When feeling tired, chunk steps so that they are smaller or simpler

	PRIORITIZE your tasks
☐	**Address emotional avoidance** ▪ Notice what feelings or thoughts might be causing you to avoid work and address it (e.g., remind yourself of your strengths, solicit support from friends or family)
☐	Set and write down 1–3 specific goals for a work session
☐	Set timers to avoid losing track of time
☐	**Take advantage of "time cracks"** ▪ While waiting for your next class to begin, you might check your email or review notes
☐	**Take timebound study breaks** ▪ Use a timer, a song, or a pre-laid walking route
	BREAK DOWN assignments into steps
☐	**Write out the steps of a large project** ▪ Estimate the time each step will take ▪ If a step feels too big, make it smaller!
☐	**Use the Pomodoro technique** ▪ Work in focused intervals of 25 minutes followed by a short 5-minute break ▪ Take a longer break after completing four 25-minute intervals
☐	Schedule studying over multiple days
	REWARD YOURSELF
☐	**Apply the Premack principle** ▪ For example, "If I complete my homework, then I can spend time with my friends"
☐	(*) What are desirable activities that increase motivation for getting work done? _____ _____

7

How to Take Notes, Read, and Study Like a Pro

Chapter Overview

- Taking Notes
- Reading and Re-Reading
- Practice Makes Perfect
- Post-Chapter Activities

For many students, it isn't until arrival at college that they realize they've never truly learned how to take notes, read, or study. Often in high school, students review test material in class, are provided study guides, or are given structured notes (e.g., fill in the blanks). For others, their high levels of intelligence carried them through high school without the need for intense studying or note-taking. Therefore, for some, it may be a challenge to know *how* to effectively study when the difficulty of material increases in college. The following chapter outlines several ways students can approach studying. Like other topics discussed in this book, your teen may require more practice of these skills with academic offices on their campus, with an educational specialist or tutor, or with a mental health professional. However, the material covered in this chapter will serve as an introduction for you and your teen and to highlight some potential methods with classwork.

TAKING NOTES

In order to have class material to study from, it's important that your teen first take notes during class. During class, many students choose to try and take notes verbatim (i.e., writing word for word what the professor is saying). Taking notes in this manner is challenging, especially true if the instructor speaks quickly. In addition to the logistical difficulties associated with verbatim note-taking, it is typically less effective in terms of comprehension. Verbatim note-taking can, in some cases, be helpful if your teen plans to thoroughly read through all of their notes multiple times. However, the research is mixed on how effective this approach is.

Generative note-taking seems to have the most support. This consists of summarizing, paraphrasing, and organizing, or outlining notes. This strategy may be helpful with retaining information and allows the note-taker to more thoroughly engage with the material. It may be difficult to organize or outline notes in the moment (e.g., while sitting in class). One option is for students to review notes at the end of each day (or week) and re-organize or paraphrase material. Electronic note-taking (i.e., taking notes on a computer) can help with this process. Alternatively, your teen may opt to draw a diagram or make a visual representation of their notes. These sorts of activities require your teen to engage with material on a deeper level and thus may increase comprehension.

Learning to take comprehensive notes may be challenging and may require work with a professional. As students are developing their note-taking skills, they may miss material in lecture. In other words, they may have trouble keeping up with what their professor is saying. There are several supports that students may take advantage of to aid in their note-taking abilities (which may need to be accessed through academic accommodations). The first is through re-listening or re-watching lectures that are provided by the instructor. Many instructors will upload copies of the lecture to the online course platform. However, not all professors record their lectures in this manner, and students may need to request academic accommodations for the ability to audio record lectures. Similarly, students may request an academic accommodation of getting a peer note-taker to provide supplemental notes. More information on these accommodations can be found in Chapter 12.

READING AND RE-READING

The first step to studying is completing the assigned reading in the first place. Reading the textbook may help to supplement material covered in lectures and reinforce concepts. Before beginning reading, it may be helpful for your teen to break down a lengthy chapter or text into more manageable pieces. This might consist of setting a goal of reading a certain number of pages or sections of a chapter. It may be helpful to revisit the material and post-chapter activities in Chapter 5 with your teen.

Once reading goals have been identified, it's important to approach the reading in a productive and efficient way. When reading a textbook, it is most helpful for students to actively read. This could consist of highlighting passages that are of most importance or taking notes in the margins. Students can also opt to take notes in the margins or supplement notes taken in class with information from the textbook. Alternatively, students can take separate notes as they read through their textbook readings. These strategies may help with retaining course material. Re-reading material may be effective when studying for a test that requires memorization; however, it's less effective if material must be integrated or applied.

PRACTICE MAKES PERFECT

The use of flash cards is one self-testing strategy that has shown great benefit for retrieving information. Students can put a term or phrase on one side of a flash card and its definition or explanation on the other. This technique has been shown to be effective for several reasons. First, flash cards require the learner to organize material (allowing for deeper engagement). In order to study with flash cards, one has to make the flash cards, which is an act of studying in itself. After making these flash cards, it's important that the learner takes adequate time studying them and ideally spreading this study over time. It's important that the learner takes breaks and does not just engage in one prolonged study period with flash cards. Additionally, it's important that flash cards aren't removed or considered mastered until the learner identifies the flashcard correctly several times. This type of self-assessment has been shown to be effective in retaining detailed information but has been less helpful at integrating and applying information.

Another effective, active study strategy is completing practice problems. Testing one's knowledge through practice exams, past exams, or past homework assignments will test for comprehension of material. Alternatively, studying with a classmate and quizzing each other on material could be helpful at recalling knowledge. However, it would be important to ensure that a study mate will be an effective accountability partner and not a distraction (see Chapter 6). These may be helpful tools in determining if one is ready for the upcoming test or quiz.

There are many different ways that students can approach studying. It's also likely that these different techniques could be more or less helpful based on the course, the type of information being learned, and the type of assessment (e.g., quiz, test). Therefore, being familiar with a wide range of techniques will best set your teen up for success as they prepare for college assessments.

POST-CHAPTER ACTIVITIES

The worksheets following this chapter will focus on study strategies and reading strategies for your teen with ADHD. As with other chapters, these post-chapter activities may require multiple discussions. On the "Study Strategies for ADHD" worksheet, you and your teen should list the current study strategies they use and how effective or ineffective they are. You and your teen should also review the listed study and note-taking strategies. In addition to reviewing study strategies, the "Reading Strategies for ADHD" worksheet will outline tips and tricks for your teen effectively getting through assigned reading for class. You and your teen should complete the questions to guide thinking and review the reading strategies.

Remember to mark off the completion of this chapter and the corresponding worksheets on the "Preparing for College Checklist" (see Chapter 1). Be sure to have your teen save a picture of the completed worksheets in the designated spot on their phone or computer.

Study Strategies for ADHD

Studying and note-taking can pose challenges for adults with ADHD. Use this worksheet to gain insight into your current habits and enhance these skills. **First, consider what study and note-taking strategies you currently use. Then, in the "Study Strategies Bank," check the corresponding box of strategies that you have tried or find appealing. Place them on the scale from "ineffective" to "effective."**

What study strategies do you currently use (e.g., studying the night before, re-reading notes, taking practice tests)? **How ineffective or effective are the strategies you currently use?** List them in the figure below.

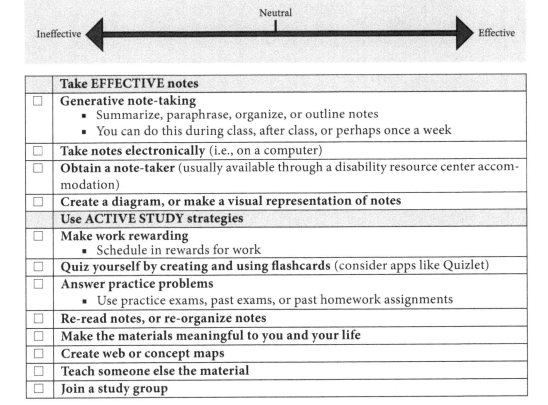

	Take EFFECTIVE notes
☐	**Generative note-taking** • Summarize, paraphrase, organize, or outline notes • You can do this during class, after class, or perhaps once a week
☐	**Take notes electronically** (i.e., on a computer)
☐	**Obtain a note-taker** (usually available through a disability resource center accommodation)
☐	**Create a diagram, or make a visual representation of notes**
	Use ACTIVE STUDY strategies
☐	**Make work rewarding** • Schedule in rewards for work
☐	**Quiz yourself by creating and using flashcards** (consider apps like Quizlet)
☐	**Answer practice problems** • Use practice exams, past exams, or past homework assignments
☐	**Re-read notes, or re-organize notes**
☐	**Make the materials meaningful to you and your life**
☐	**Create web or concept maps**
☐	**Teach someone else the material**
☐	**Join a study group**

Reading Strategies for ADHD

Reading can be difficult for adults with ADHD for many reasons, including difficulties with focusing, working memory, sitting still, managing time, and managing distractions. If you want to improve these skills, some of the strategies listed below may be helpful! **Check a box next to 1–2 strategies below that you would be interested in trying for one week. Answer the questions marked with a star (★) to guide your thinking.**

	Make reading ACCESSIBLE

☐	**Choose the format of your reading materials**
	
	 (★) Do you prefer digital or printed reading materials?_____
	
	 (★) If you prefer digital materials...
	  ... how accessible and organized are your virtual folders? _____
	  ... are you using a program that makes annotations and note-taking easy? _____
	
	 (★) If you prefer printed materials, are they printed and kept in a single, visible space (e.g., a folder on your desk)? _____

☐	**Read in a comfortable space** (★) Where do you do your best reading (e.g., home, library)? _____
☐	**Schedule specific times and hours to read** (★) When do you do your best reading (e.g., morning, afternoon)?_____ (★) How much text can you read before focusing feels too effortful (e.g., one paragraph, one chapter, one page)?_____
	Utilize ACTIVE READING
☐	**Use pens or highlighters to:** • Track words • Note interesting facts • Identify important claims made by the author • Make revisiting important content later on an easier task

☐	Read out loud
☐	Write notes (especially *questions*) in the margins of a text or on a separate piece of paper
☐	Quiz yourself on sections before moving on
☐	Draw pictures of what you read to better understand a concept
☐	When possible, read content that interests you (★) What type of content is easy for you to read? _____ (★) What type of content is difficult for you to read? _____
☐	Summarize the entirety of or a section of what you read using bullet points • Turn section headers into questions, and then answer them using your summary
	Elicit a SOCIAL ASSIST
☐	Read beside a friend
☐	Discuss the material with a friend
	Manage feelings of OVERWHELM
☐	Acknowledge what about reading is stressful for you • Remember: reading involves many complex steps. **It is normal for many people with ADHD to find it challenging.**
☐	Take timebound breaks
☐	**Schedule reading sessions** across multiple days
☐	**Reward yourself for reading a specified amount of text** (e.g., two sentences, a page) (★) What might you reward your success with (e.g., candy, a 2-minute song break)? _____
☐	**Reward yourself for reading for a specified amount of time** (e.g., 5 minutes, 30 minutes) (★) What might you reward your success with (e.g., candy, a 2-minute song break)? _____

PART III

Preparing the Application and Selecting the Right School

8

Selecting the Right School

Chapter Overview

- General Criteria for Choosing a School
- College Specialties
- Post-Chapter Activities

There are thousands of two-year and four-year colleges and universities in the United States, and this number increases sixfold when we consider postsecondary institutions abroad. So how do you and your teen decide on the right place for them to take the next step in their academic journey? And how does ADHD play a role in that decision-making process? This chapter will outline a variety of considerations you and your teen should weigh when ultimately deciding which institution your teen plans to attend.

It is important to note which factors bear more or less weight in the college decision-making process—and this may differ from family to family. This chapter and associated activities should be used as a guide rather than an exact formula. The first section is applicable to all students whereas the following sections will focus on topics specific to teens with ADHD. It's important to discuss these considerations both prior to your teen applying to college (e.g., when developing their list of schools to apply to) as well as when your teen decides which school to enroll in. It may be helpful for you to discuss potential universities using the following groups: "needs" (features that are required for selecting a school), "wants" (features in a university that are desired by you and your teen but aren't the most important or necessary—a wish list), and "dealbreakers" (features that would rule a university off your list).

GENERAL CRITERIA FOR CHOOSING A SCHOOL

It goes without saying that for the majority of families there are several factors that play a major role or are the deciding factors in determining where their teen will study: academics, location, and financial aid.

Academics

The first decision you and your teen may want to discuss is whether you and your teen feel that initially attending a two-year college (i.e., community college) and transferring to a four-year university would be more suitable compared to immediately entering a four-year institution. For some students, obtaining their associate's degree at a two-year institution before transferring to receive their bachelor's degree has many advantages. First, it may help teens more slowly acclimate to the academic demands of college. For many teens the transition from high school to college comes with an increase in academic demands (e.g., having to manage a more difficult course load, less oversight from parents and teachers, balancing academics and responsibilities of daily living). Therefore, getting their footing in a two-year college where the academic demands may be somewhat less challenging compared to a four-year university may be the right decision for some families. Typically, the per credit cost is also less expensive at two-year colleges compared to four-year institutions. Some students may opt to fulfill prerequisite (or introductory) courses at a two-year institution and apply to transfer to a four-year after receiving their associate's degree.

If you and your teen decide that applying to a four-year university is the best course of action, one of the most important considerations is choosing a school that offers a major in what your teen is interested in studying. Though many schools will have a great deal of overlap in the majors and minors that they offer, certain universities might offer unique majors, extensive study abroad programs, built-in or required internships or "co-op" experiences, or accelerated bachelor's degree to graduate degree programs—all of which may be important pieces of information in the decision process. Certain schools may be highly ranked in a certain area given faculty expertise or courses offered. This type of information is found in places like the university or college website or on national ranking lists found online. Alternatively, students may be undecided on what they want to study and therefore, may want to consider selecting a school that has a wide variety of majors that may appeal to them.

The last facet of academics that families should consider is the likelihood of admittance into schools. Experts suggest that students apply to a range of 4 to 15 colleges and universities, depending on their admittance rate. When developing a list of schools to apply to, you and your teen should consider the average grade point average (GPA), average standardized test scores (if applicable), and admissions rates. These statistics are typically published on each school's admissions website. It's recommended that your teen applies to several "safety," "target," and "reach" schools. Safety schools are schools in which your teen's GPA or test scores exceed the average admittance statistics or where the admittance rate is high. Target schools are schools in which your teen's academic achievement or test scores are roughly equivalent to the average admittance statistics. Reach schools are schools where your teen's GPA or standardized test scores fall at or below the school's average or the acceptance rate is fairly low. Students should consider submitting the most applications to target schools, with several safety or reach schools in the mix. This will offer your teen the best chances for not only being accepted to a university but to have several schools to choose from! Ultimately, the number of schools your teen applies to will depend on the distribution of safety, target, and reach schools, as well as financial matters. Each application submission costs approximately $30–$90, so deciding upon the number of submissions should be balanced with having the greatest likelihood of acceptance while staying within a predetermined budget.

You and your teen may be thinking, "That's a lot of schools to look into!" Though that's true, there are other factors that will limit the search. Other information such as financials and location, as well as factors related to ADHD, are outlined through the remainder of the chapter and will help to narrow down you and your teen's search.

Location

One factor that may narrow down the college search is the location of the school. Some families may decide that it is important for their teen to live at home while attending school. Therefore, applying to schools that are within a reasonable commuting distance will narrow down options. For other students, living away from home (i.e., living in the dorms on campus, living in an off-campus apartment) may be an option. You and your teen will need to discuss what proximity is ideal (e.g., within driving distance, within the same state, on the same coast of the country), or if there are no geographical restrictions.

It may also be helpful to consider location in terms of the social support readily available by a particular university. As described in Chapter 14, "Dealing with Depression," college students with ADHD are at higher risk for experiencing depression than their peers without ADHD. Loneliness and lack of support may also contribute to the presence of depression. Therefore, having immediate family, extended family, or a built-in friend network could help ease the transition to college for students with ADHD, especially those who may struggle with forming friendships or those who need additional support. For instance, your teen may want to consider being within driving distance of their family home. Alternatively, your teen may want to consider locations where there is extended family in the community nearby the university campus or a university in which one of your teen's friends or family members is attending. These geographical considerations may help to narrow the focus to a certain area of the state or country.

Finances

Finances are an important consideration for the majority of families. In addition to helping to inform whether teens attend a two-year or four-year college, finances also may inform where teens enroll. The cost of tuition, room and board (if not living at home), books, a computer, and living expenses are all things that need to be considered when selecting a school. It is important for families to be transparent about who and how the college education will be covered. This could include funding from one (or many) of the following forms: (1) parental support, (2) student support (employment), (3) university scholarships, (4) outside scholarships, (5) federal work study programs, (6) federal student loans, (7) private student loans, and (8) armed forces Reserve Officer Training Corps (ROTC) scholarships. It is important for both parents and students to have a clear understanding of what the cost of attendance of each college option will be and how this will be paid for. Students should understand the consequences of attending a school that is more expensive, where less financial support (e.g., scholarships) was provided, or where room and board would be necessary (i.e., going to school away from home). The solution may be that your teen will need to work a full-time or part-time job to support themselves, take out student loans from one or more institutions, or apply for additional scholarship opportunities.

COLLEGE SPECIALTIES

After outlining some of the general criteria for selecting a university, diving into the details may help to narrow down your teen's list of potential schools. You and your teen may want to consider class size and specialty resources available at each school to guide in your decision-making process.

Class Size

Class sizes should be an important consideration for all students, but may be something especially critical for families with a teen with ADHD to especially think about. Many teens are accustomed to relatively small class sizes in high school where they receive a good deal of individual attention from teachers. However, there is a wide variety of class sizes and types across colleges. For example, some classes (e.g., introductory classes, lecture-style courses) may have enrollments of one hundred students or more and be held in large lecture halls. In these courses, it may be more difficult for professors to give individualized attention to students (e.g., reaching out to students who appear to be struggling or who have missing assignments). This likely requires students to be more proactive with reaching out to professors or teaching assistants for help. It also may not be clear to professors if students are attending class regularly in large lecture halls with many students, which means students will need to be self-motivated to attend class as their absence may not be noticed.

Smaller class sizes may have several advantages for students with ADHD. First, in smaller classes, students may receive more individualized attention, and their presence and participation are more apparent. Smaller class sizes may help students feel more comfortable asking questions during class or approaching a faculty member or teaching assistant with requests for help with the material. This is not to suggest that students with ADHD cannot flourish in large, lecture-style classes. It just may be that students with ADHD need to be especially proactive with learning skills (mentioned in Chapters 5–7) and using resources (described in Chapters 10, 11, and 13).

Class size is something that can be found in a variety of places. Most universities post average class size statistics on their admissions website. Another helpful metric that can be found on most admissions websites is the student to faculty ratio, or the number of students on campus compared to the number of faculty members. For example, a 10:1 student to faculty ratio means that there are 10 times as many students as faculty members (or for every 10 students, there is 1 faculty member). Though these metrics are certainly helpful, they are just an average across the entire university. It may be helpful to discuss more specific statistics with tour guides or program administrators within your student's anticipated major. It may be that within a certain major (e.g., English, creative writing, foreign languages), small class size is typical, whereas other majors (e.g., sciences, technology, engineering, mathematics or STEM), the norm may be large lecture classes with supplemental laboratory and discussion sections where students meet in smaller groups. If class size is an important consideration, it could be helpful to know what the typical class size looks like in your teen's potential major (in addition to metrics on the university as a whole).

Specialty Services for ADHD and Neurodevelopmental Difficulties

On the majority of university campuses (if not all), there is some degree of academic or mental health resources. These resources are explained in more detail in Chapter 12, but typically consist of disability resource centers (where students obtain academic accommodations) and counseling centers (where students obtain brief mental health counseling). However, there are some colleges and universities that offer specialty services that may be of interest to you and your teen. This may consist of peer mentoring programs, specialty ADHD clinics, and programs that provide assistance with organization, time management, and learning and study skills. There are also institutions that have been designed specifically for college students with ADHD, autism, or learning difficulties. If these types of resources are crucial for selecting a college, it is important to explore what types of specialty resources are available to students on campus. Though not exhaustive, the following list of schools offer specialty services on-campus for students with ADHD, learning difficulties, or neurodevelopmental conditions:

- American University: Learning Services Program
- Augsburg University: Center for Learning and Accessible Student Services (CLASS)
- Beacon College: College created to help students with learning disabilities and ADHD
- Curry College: Program of Advancement Learning
- Davis & Elkins College: Supported Learning Program (SLP)
- Dean College: Arch Learning Community (ALC)
- Hofstra University: Program for Academic Learning Skills (PALS)
- Landmark College: A college exclusively for neurodiverse students
- Lynn University: Institute for Achievement and Learning (IAL)
- Marist College: Learning Support Program (LSP)
- McDaniel College: Student Accessibility Support Services
- Mitchell College: Thames Academy transition program
- Northeastern University: Learning Disabilities
- Rutgers University: ACCESS Program
- University of Arizona: Strategic Alternative Learning Techniques Center
- University of Denver: Learning Effectiveness Program
- University of Illinois, Chicago: SUCCEEDS ADHD Clinic
- University of Iowa: Realizing Educational and Career Hopes (REACH)
- University of Maryland, College Park: SUCCEEDS ADHD Clinic; SIGNA Autism Clinic
- University of the Ozarks: Jones Learning Center
- West Virginia Wesleyan College: Mentor Advantage Program

Given that this list is not exhaustive, it could be helpful to contact the disability resource center at schools where your teen has interest in applying to get more detailed information. You should ask them about any specialty services for college students with ADHD or general services that help support students in the transition from high school to college (e.g., summer programs, seminars in students' first semester).

POST-CHAPTER ACTIVITIES

There are several conversations and tasks associated with selecting a college or university. Therefore, it may take several discussions around this topic to progress through these post-chapter activities. First, it's important for you and your teen to discuss finances and how they will realistically cover the costs of both applications to college and college itself. With your teen, complete the "Application Budget" and "College Budget" worksheets. Knowing how students and their families plan to pay for college may help guide the additional steps in searching for schools. After discussing finances, it's time for you and your teen to discuss the wants, needs, and dealbreakers using the "Choosing a College" worksheet. After these conversations, it's time for you and your teen to begin exploring colleges and entering data into the "School Data" tables to compile a list of possible schools to apply to.

Remember to mark off the completion of this chapter and the corresponding worksheets on the "Preparing for College Checklist" (see Chapter 1). Be sure to have your teen save a picture of the completed worksheets in the designated spot on their phone or computer.

Application Budget

Money is an important consideration when applying to college. Use this worksheet to estimate how much you would ideally spend and the maximum you would be able to spend on an expense (e.g., application fees). Then, calculate your ideal amount and sources of income.

	COSTS	NOTES
Standardized Testing (if applicable)	IDEAL: $_____ MAXIMUM: $_____	
Application Fees	IDEAL: $_____ MAXIMUM: $_____	
College Visits	IDEAL: $_____ MAXIMUM: $_____	
Other Costs	IDEAL: $_____ MAXIMUM: $_____	
	INCOME	**NOTES**
Self-Employment	IDEAL: $_____	
Family Contribution (if possible)	IDEAL: $_____	
Additional Funding	IDEAL: $_____	Preferred source of funding: o Local, state, or national scholarships o Other: _____

(TOTAL INCOME: $_____) - (TOTAL COST: $_____) = $_____

Selecting the Right School

College Budget

Money is also an important consideration when attending college. Use this worksheet to estimate how much you would ideally spend and the maximum you would be able to spend on an expense (e.g., tuition across four years). Then, calculate your ideal amount and sources of income.

	COSTS	NOTES
Tuition	IDEAL: $_____ MAXIMUM: $_____	
Room and Board	IDEAL: $_____ MAXIMUM: $_____	
Meal Plan	IDEAL: $_____ MAXIMUM: $_____	
Other Costs	IDEAL: $_____ MAXIMUM: $_____	This estimate includes: o Books and supplies o Fees o Insurance o Transportation o Other: _____
	INCOME	**NOTES**
Student Loans	IDEAL: $_____ MAXIMUM: $_____	Preferred types of loans: o Federal o Private o Other: _____
College Funding	IDEAL: $_____	Preferred source of funding: o College scholarships o Federal work-study o Local, state, or national scholarships o Other: _____
Self-Employment	IDEAL: $_____	Type of student employment: o Full time o Part time
Family Contribution (if possible)	IDEAL: $_____	
(TOTAL INCOME: $_____) - (TOTAL COST: $_____) = $_____		

Choosing a College

Choosing the right college can feel overwhelming. It may be helpful to use this table to categorize your considerations into needs, wants, and dealbreakers. "Needs" are essential features that a college must have to be a real option for you. "Wants" are desirable attributes that while not necessary, would enhance your experience. "Dealbreakers" are features of a college that would immediately disqualify it from your list.

Academics	▶ What kind of institution should I attend (e.g., two-year program, four-year program)? ▶ What majors and courses should my college have available to me? ▶ How rigorous should coursework be—should my college be highly ranked in a certain area?	
Needs	Wants	Dealbreakers

College Specialties	▶ Should my college have built-in or required internship or co-op experiences? ▶ Am I interested in an extensive study abroad program? ▶ How large do I want the average class size to be? ▶ What mental health, academic, or ADHD-specific resources do I want to be available? ▶ Any other special considerations?	
Needs	Wants	Dealbreakers

Location	▶ Should my college be in commuting distance? ▶ If not commuting, how close should my college be to family?	
Needs	Wants	Dealbreakers

Financial Aid	▶ Given the costs I expect to incur at college, what kind of funding do I need from the college (i.e., college scholarships, ROTC scholarships, access to federal work-study programs)?	
Needs	Wants	Dealbreakers

School Data

School Name	Location	# of Undergrads Enrolled	Student: Faculty Ratio	Common App Available (Y/N)	Essays Required	SAT/ACT Required?	# letters of Rec Required	Accept Rate
Example: University of Illinois Chicago	Chicago, IL	22,107	18:1	Yes	Common App; UIC career essay	Optional	2	78.7%

Application Due Date	Application Fee	Tuition and Fees Cost	Room and Board Cost	ADHD/Learning Resources Available?	Pros	Cons
4/5/24	$70	$16,518 per year	$14,400	SUCCEEDS Clinic	Diverse student body; health science major	Less traditional campus, in the city

School Name	Location	# of Undergrads Enrolled	Student: Faculty Ratio	Common App Available (Y/N)	Essays Required	SAT/ACT Required?	# letters of Rec Required	Accept Rate

Application Due Date	Application Fee	Tuition and Fees Cost	Room and Board Cost	ADHD/Learning Resources Available?	Pros	Cons

9
Submitting the Application

Chapter Outline

- Application Forms
- College Essays
- Standardized Tests
- Letters of Recommendation
- Early Decision and Early Acceptance Options
- Miscellaneous Necessities
- Post-Chapter Activities

There are many components to submitting a successful college application: forms, essays, standardized tests, and letters of recommendations, to name a few. Before submitting the application, it's important to first understand what your teen wants in a college. Following Chapter 5, you and your teen will hopefully have decided what it is they're looking for when it comes to selecting a school. The last chapter also tasked you and your teen with selecting a range of 4–15 schools that fall into safety, target, and reach categories. Once your teen has the makings of a list of colleges to apply to, it's time to shift gears and work on the application itself. This chapter will outline the various tasks (and when to complete them) in terms of applying for college.

APPLICATION FORMS

With any application, there are forms that need to be completed online. These forms typically consist of demographic information that needs to be entered about your teen (e.g., name, date of birth, address, nationality) and your teen's education and extracurricular activities (e.g., high school information, community involvement). By entering your teen's high school information into application portals, it will trigger an email to the high school to provide grades and academic standing for your teen. Though entering all this demographic information may be considered one of the easiest parts of the college application, it can be quite time-consuming. However, the Common App was developed to simplify the college application process and reduce some of the logistical burdens. In addition to offering a college selection search engine (discussed in Chapter 9), it also allows applicants to enter their application information in one system and send it to their selected schools. Over 1,000 schools in the United States accept the Common App. Students create a profile, add desired universities to the list, upload essays, and enter letter of recommendation writers' information (they will receive an email to submit their letter through the Common App). This saves students a good deal of time by holding and organizing all this information in one centralized location. Though many schools accept the Common App, not all the schools on your teen's list may do so. Therefore, there still may be some schools that require you to enter this information in a school-specific portal.

COLLEGE ESSAYS

Unlike the application forms, the college essay is considered the most difficult for many high schoolers. In some cases, students may need to write multiple essays. Therefore, it's crucial for your teen to begin this part of the application early so that there is sufficient time for writing one or more essays as well as time to read and revise it before submitting. The writing prompts may be similar across institutions (or unique to a particular school), so it is important for you and your teen to explore each school's requirements well in advance of the submission deadline.

If submitting an application to a school through the Common App portal, your teen will be asked to write one personal essay from a list of possibilities. These prompts include things like (1) discussing a talent or accomplishment, (2) describing a challenge you've overcome, (3) writing about a time you've questioned a belief or idea, (4) expressing something you're grateful for, (5) writing about a topic that you are interested in, or (6) sharing an essay you have previously written and are proud of. For schools that do not accept the Common App, prompts are often quite similar.

In addition to the personal essay portion, schools may require one or more supplemental essays or short answer responses. The prompts for these writing supplements vary widely from school to school, but may include describing why and how a student is interested in their university or a specific major, how the student will explore the community at their university, a list of books a student has enjoyed outside of coursework, or addressing one of the prompts similar to the ones listed above in regard to the Common App. Typically, more competitive schools require more supplemental writing prompts. Studying each school's requirements is important to ensuring a student submits a complete application.

The college essays are an opportunity for your teen to introduce themselves to the admissions committee at an institution. Admissions committees review thousands of applications, and this is a place where your teen can make their application stand out. Therefore, it's important your teen has plenty of time to write their essays. Not only should your teen allocate enough time to create the writing assignments, but they should make sure they have enough time to also have a trusted adult read through their materials (e.g., parent, older sibling, teacher) and revise accordingly.

STANDARDIZED TESTS

After the COVID-19 pandemic, the future of standardized tests remains uncertain. In the past, students were required to take either the SAT (Standardized Achievement Test) or the ACT (American College Testing). However, during the COVID-19 pandemic, health and safety guidelines prohibited the administration of these tests. After the discontinuation of COVID-19 restrictions, the standardized testing requirements were not universally reinstated. Many schools have made submitting standardized test scores optional (at least for the time being). Other schools are beginning to require standardized test scores as part of the admissions portfolio. Therefore, it is also important to decide upon a list of schools to apply to and determine whether taking standardized tests are needed.

If taking the test is required for schools your teen is applying to, it is important to plan as early as possible. It may be important for your teen to understand their strengths and difficulties on the test. For example, in completing a practice test, students may come to realize that they're a superstar on the math section but struggle with the verbal section, or vice versa, or that they need to study all of the sections. Completing a practice test early will allow your teen ample time to study if needed. It is important that your teen takes the practice test as if it's the real one (e.g., without using notes, within the allotted time frame, in a quiet space) to get an accurate reading on their current performance.

Once you and your teen understand what areas they need to study, you both can decide on a preparation plan. There are many options (which will also depend on your family's budget). First, all students should take advantage of freely available practice tests online. If additional tests are necessary, your family could also consider purchasing SAT or ACT preparatory materials from any retailer that sells books. These books can help with providing practice problems, study strategies, common vocabulary words seen on these tests, and practice tests. Though self-guided study can certainly be an effective way to prepare for standardized testing, it does require diligence and a plan on the part of the student (and parent to enforce it). It could be helpful to create a routine (e.g., schedule a specific day or time every week) in terms of studying with a finish line or test date in mind. An alternative to these self-guided strategies is hiring an SAT or ACT tutor. Though this comes with benefits (e.g., someone to keep your teen accountable, individualized lesson plans), it certainly comes with a cost. Therefore, the type of learning style and budget will help determine which study plan is best suited for your teen.

Aside from having ample time to study, beginning standardized testing preparation early is important given that students may wish to take the SAT or ACT more than once. There is virtually no limit to the number of times your teen can take the SAT; the ACT can only be taken by a student 12 times, but most students only retake the exam once or twice. However, the SAT is only offered about 7 times per year and registration needs to occur about a month before the test date. It also takes about 2–4 weeks for students to receive their SAT or ACT scoring results. Therefore, beginning this process early will allow for your teen to have ample time to take a test, receive their test score, register for another test, and take it a second (or third) time if needed. A quick note on taking standardized tests: most universities elect to use "super-scoring," in which the highest score on each section of the test (regardless of which test date) is used to create a composite. For example, a student may have scored higher on the math section the first time they took the SAT but scored highest on the verbal section during their second attempt. Super-scoring means these two high scores are combined, resulting in the highest composite score. This ensures there is no penalty for taking a standardized test more than once.

Each administration of a standardized test comes with a cost, so it's important your teen approach the test seriously. If cost is a barrier, there are fee waivers for standardized tests that can be obtained through your teen's school counselor or by applying to the college board directly (SAT only; https://satsuite.collegeboard.org/sat/registration/fee-waivers). Students are eligible if they are enrolled in the 11th or 12th grade, are taking the test within the United States or territories, and one of the following criteria: (1) enrolled in a federal free or reduced-price lunch program, (2) enrolled in a program for economically disadvantaged students (e.g., GEAR UP), (3) resides in foster home, (4) family receives low-income public assistance or lives in federally subsidized public housing, (5) family's total annual income is at or below the USDA level for free or reduced-price lunches (https://www.fns.usda.gov/cn/income-eligibility-guidelines).

LETTERS OF RECOMMENDATION

Letters of recommendation are an important component to your teen's college application. Typically, universities require a recommendation form or letter from a high school guidance counselor as well as from one of their teachers. These letters or forms should be used to highlight your teen's strengths in the classroom, involvement in extracurricular activities, and goals and ambitions. Therefore, it is important that students identify writers who can speak to these areas. Students may select a teacher of a class that they performed particularly well in or a teacher with whom they completed extracurricular activities. Some universities allow for additional recommendations from an arts teacher, mentor, clergy member, coach, or employer. These individuals may be able to speak to your teen's interest, character, determination, and positive qualities outside the traditional classroom. If using the Common App, invitations for letter writers will be sent through their system. Alternatively, at individual schools, letter writers provide contact information (e.g., email addresses are entered by the student) and invitations are sent electronically.

EARLY DECISION AND EARLY ACCEPTANCE OPTIONS

Outside of the traditional application timeline (i.e., being notified of admissions decisions in March or April) there are several options in which students are notified earlier. However, these paths also require students to submit their application by an earlier deadline (early November) compared to the regular application deadline (December or January). The first early path is through "early decision." Early decision offers students the opportunity to be notified earlier of admissions decisions, but is a binding agreement (i.e., if applicants are accepted then they are committed to attending that school). This can be helpful because the admissions rates tend to be slightly higher with early decision than in the standard application process. The downside is that a student's acceptance is bound to that school regardless of the financial aid offered. Some schools will offer two early decision deadlines, with the first having a due date of November and the second due in December or January. Both are binding, but the second option offers applicants more time to complete their application and visit a campus. Therefore, if your teen has a clear first choice school and financial aid is not a concern, early decision will offer the best odds of acceptance.

"Early action" is the second path, and is not binding. Early action requires students to submit their application before the regular admissions deadline but may increase a students' chances of acceptance and allow them to be notified of an admissions decision early. However, early action is less common than early decision, and offered at fewer schools. Therefore, if your teen completes their applications by November and a school offers early action, it may be beneficial to apply through this program since it increases chances of acceptance without it being binding.

MISCELLANEOUS NECESSITIES

In addition to the typical necessities of college applications, your teen may have additional requirements depending on the school or major they are applying to. For example, students applying for music or performing arts will likely have to prepare for an audition. This may consist of practicing audition pieces and being prepared to sight read music. For students applying to art or design school, their application process may involve putting together a portfolio of their work and scheduling an interview to review the contents with an admissions representative.

Some schools (typically highly selective or Ivy League universities) offer or may require an interview with an alumnus or admissions representative. The goals of these interviews may vary, from providing the applicant with information about the university to evaluating the applicant. In some cases, these interviews may be recommended while in others it is required. Some schools may reach out to students if they qualify for an interview, whereas others may require your teen to schedule an optional interview if they are interested. Regardless, it is important for you and your teen to investigate whether there are additional components or interviews required or recommended for any of the schools that they are applying to.

POST-CHAPTER ACTIVITIES

After reading about the necessary components to your teen's college application through this chapter, please review and complete the "Application Checklist" worksheet with your teen to arrive at a mutually agreed upon timeline for completing their college applications. Following Chapter 8, your teen and you should have constructed a list of potential schools to apply to. At this point, you and your teen should begin to narrow down potential options and enter the final list of schools on the "Selected Schools" worksheet.

Remember to mark off the completion of this chapter and the corresponding worksheets on the "Preparing for College Checklist" (see Chapter 1). Be sure to have your teen save a picture of the completed worksheets in the designated spot on their phone or computer.

Application Checklist

Task	Scheduled Deadline
☐ Select Schools	_____
☐ Take Standardized Test (if needed)	_____
☐ Identify Letter Writers:	_____

    1. _____

    2. _____

    3. _____

☐ Write Essay

☐ _____   _____

☐ _____   _____

☐ _____   _____

☐ Fill Out Applications Online   _____

☐ Submit Applications (by due date)

☐ _____

☐ _____

☐ Celebrate!

Selected Schools

Safety Schools

1. _____
2. _____
3. _____
4. _____
5. _____

Target Schools

1. _____
2. _____
3. _____
4. _____
5. _____

Reach Schools

1. _____
2. _____
3. _____
4. _____
5. _____

Selected Schools

Safety Schools	Admission Decision
1.	
2.	
3.	
4.	
5.	

Target Schools	Admission Decision
6.	
7.	
8.	
9.	
10.	

Reach Schools	Admission Decision
11.	
12.	
13.	
14.	
15.	

PART IV

Getting to Know Your Teen's Campus and Classes

10

Hiding in Plain Sight

Campus Resources

Chapter Outline

- Academic Resources
- Physical and Mental Health Resources and Community Support
- Logistical Resources
- Post-Chapter Activities

Though many of these resources have been mentioned in previous chapters of this book, this chapter will outline the academic, mental health, and logistical resources that are available on university campuses. Despite their availability, students may not be aware of these resources. Though new student orientation and student affairs expos are great ways to learn about the numerous supports offered to students, this chapter will highlight the general resources that most (if not all) schools offer. The post-chapter activity will serve as a way for you and your teen to explore where and how your teen can access these resources at their university.

ACADEMIC RESOURCES

Universities are equipped with numerous resources on campus to assist in students' academic success. These include though are not limited to academic advising, academic accommodations, office hours, tutoring, and writing assistance.

Academic Advising

Chapter 12 will highlight the importance of academic advising in relation to deciding upon course loads and schedules. Though this is certainly one of the primary domains of advisors, they are helpful across additional academic areas as well. For instance, academic advisors help students decide upon a major (should they be undecided) or change majors at any point during their college years. They often recommend classes (or electives) that might be in line with students' interests. Should students struggle with a class and need to withdraw or take an incomplete (i.e., finish course after the semester ends), academic advisors can walk students through the process and help file necessary paperwork. Should a student need to discuss any difficulties they are experiencing in a course, an academic advisor could be a sounding board for these issues. Academic advisors are also a great referral source for other resources for students to use on campus. Students should spend time getting to know their academic advisor outside of just required meetings for course registration.

Disability Resource Center

An additional academic resource that has been previously discussed in this book is academic accommodations, which are accessed through the college's disability resource center (see Chapter 12). Academic accommodations are modifications made to an academic experience (e.g., private testing, extended test time, flexible deadlines, excused absences) to combat educational difficulties that may impede success. Though the disability resource center is essential to obtaining accommodations, this resource center can be helpful for students throughout their time at college. For instance, if students need to amend their accommodations (i.e., add an additional accommodation), meeting with the disability resource is necessary. If students encounter difficulties using their accommodations (i.e., a professor does not abide by an accommodation letter), the disability resource center can help advocate on a student's behalf. The disability resource center may also be able to link your teen with tutoring, coaching, or therapy services on campus.

Office Hours

Office hours are designated times set during the week for professors and teaching assistants (TAs) to meet with students about course content. If students can't attend these set hours, professors and TAs are typically accommodating in setting up an additional time to meet. Attending office hours is helpful for a variety of reasons. First, and most obvious, office hours are a place where students can get questions answered, course content clarified, and learn from mistakes on exams or assignments. Sometimes professors and TAs will hold exam review sessions in office hours as well. Second, office hours represent a way in which students can introduce themselves to their professors and teaching assistants. Class sizes vary at college, and in some cases a course could have as many as 150 students in it. In these large lectures, it can be difficult for a professor or teaching assistant to get to know every student on a first-name basis. Office hours are a great place to develop professional relationships with instructors on campus. This is important, because eventually students may need letters of recommendation or references for graduate school applications or a job. The more an instructor is familiar with a student, the stronger letter or reference will be. Having a stronger relationship with faculty could help open the door for additional opportunities (e.g., internships, research experiences).

Tutoring and Study Sessions

There are other venues for students to receive assistance with course material in addition to attending office hours or meetings with professors. There are several opportunities for tutoring on campus. Departments often have designated tutors for traditionally difficult courses in which they hire former students in a class to provide free assistance to current students. These sessions are generally conducted in a group format. Informal peer tutoring may be available in classes too. For instance, students in classes may organize informal study groups where they review material together. These academic resources (both formal and informal) are helpful in ensuring your teen has a solid grasp on course material.

Writing Assistance

Many college students, regardless of having ADHD, may struggle with writing assignments. There are many components to writing a successful paper and students may have trouble with any of the pieces along the way. College writing assignments, like research papers, often require students to find primary sources to support their work. For students who have not had to write a research paper before, it may be challenging to know where to find the information to support their argument in a paper and how to cite it properly. One of the best places to go for assistance with this research phase is the library. The library is not merely a building with books. Library staff can be invaluable at teaching students how and where to conduct research and find sources for their paper. Utilizing library personnel will help to make the research process easier, especially for the first writing assignment of their college career.

In addition to getting help with the research process, there are often free resources on campus that help with the writing and editing process. For example, most universities have a writing center in which there are staff members (typically undergraduate or graduate student workers) who will read through a student's assignment and provide detailed feedback. This mentoring can be used for other types of writing too (e.g., personal statements, cover letters, resumes), not just class assignments. If a student has difficulty with structuring an essay, getting started on a paper, or revising or strengthening content, the university writing center is an excellent resource to try.

PHYSICAL AND MENTAL HEALTH RESOURCES AND COMMUNITY SUPPORT

Aside from academic resources, campuses also offer many resources for student mental health, physical health, and general well-being.

Student Health Center

Should your teen need any medical attention during their time at university, the student health center is the place to go. The student health center typically addresses common concerns like infections, viruses, vaccinations and immunizations, and other issues that would be typically addressed with a primary care provider or pediatrician. Other specialty services may also be available in areas like physical therapy, radiology, lab services (e.g., blood work), reproductive and sexual health, or gender-affirming care. It may be that the university student health center partners with the university hospital system (if one exists) so that when more specialty care is needed, students will be referred to the correct hospital department. Regardless, the student health center should be your teen's first stop for any health-related concerns (unless they have a local primary care provider or pediatrician whose care they remain under).

Wellness services will often fall under the umbrella of the student health center, but at some universities these resources may fall under a separate center. Wellness services are at the intersection of mental and physical health. Universities may offer meditation sessions, stress reduction seminars, nutritional counseling or food assistance, alcohol and drug education, relationship counseling, and gender-based violence advocacy.

Mental Health Counseling

Counseling services are a standard offering at universities. Traditionally, university counseling centers will provide short-term care to help students with pressing mental health concerns. Though not a universal policy, many counseling centers place a limit on the number of therapy sessions a student can schedule per academic year. This is typically due to the high demand for counseling center sessions and there not being enough therapists to be able to offer students unlimited sessions. Services at the university counseling center traditionally are designed to be time-limited in nature and focused on one goal or crisis. If students need more intensive or long-term mental health care, the counseling center may help to refer students to mental health professionals outside of the university that accept the student's insurance. Given that the counseling center may have a waitlist, it is important for your teen to contact the counseling center as soon as possible when and if they need support. It may be a week or more before they will be seen for a therapy session (unless, of course, they are in the midst of a serious crisis). The counseling center likely also has providers that prescribe medication if warranted and if desired by your teen.

In addition to counseling centers, universities may also have a training clinic with providers being graduate students in a mental health field (e.g., clinical psychology). More specifically, if a university offers a graduate program in clinical psychology, they will often contain an in-house clinic where graduate students see patients as part of their training under the supervision of licensed clinical psychologists (their professors). This is another great option for students to receive mental health care, especially if the counseling center has a long waitlist or if your teen has maxed out the number of sessions at the counseling center. Though the clinicians are graduate students, they go through many hours of training prior to seeing patients and receive direction from supervisors. A training clinic such as this will likely be located on campus and is traditionally part of the Department of Psychology.

Finally, some universities will offer academic coaching (often by fellow undergraduate students). Individuals (typically more advanced undergraduate students) meet with students and help to provide them with skills on how to take notes, study, approach tests strategically, and manage their time. Though this peer mentorship is certainly valuable, it may be important for your teen to supplement it by working with a mental health professional.

Community Support

There are also opportunities for more informal social support on campus. Universities have a multitude of extracurricular student groups for your teen to join, whether it be Greek life (e.g., fraternities, sororities), academic in nature (e.g., pre-med, pre-dental, pre-law, Quiz Bowl), recreational (e.g., intramural or club sports), literature and performing arts (e.g., musical groups, acapella, bands, theater, poetry, improv), cultural (e.g., student run groups for students of specific racial and ethnic backgrounds, LGBTQ community, religious groups, Women in STEM), or service based (e.g., volunteering in the community). Typically, at the beginning of the fall semester (and sometimes at the beginning of the spring semester too) there is an activities fair for students to see the wide variety of student-led organizations for students to get involved in. Though your teen doesn't necessarily have to join an activity at the beginning of the semester, these fairs are excellent ways to see all their options in one place without having to find information on the internet (or elsewhere) about meeting times. Having peer support may not only help with your teen's mental health, but may also help provide structure to non–class time and increase your teen's social network.

There may also be university-run offices or centers for students to get involved in. Students could get involved with the admissions office to become a campus tour guide. Students could opt to join the Reserve Officer Training Corps (ROTC), which provides structure and scholarships. The campus might also have cultural centers, offices, or religious spaces for students of various racial, ethnic, cultural, gender, or religious groups.

LOGISTICAL RESOURCES

In addition to the academic, mental and physical health, and community support, there are other miscellaneous individuals on campus that help with logistical support.

Information Technology (IT) Office

The IT office helps to address technological concerns. If students are having difficulty accessing wireless internet on campus or are having difficulty accessing course content on online platforms (e.g., Blackboard, Canvas), the IT office can help to troubleshoot. Additionally, if a student's computer breaks, they may be able to offer technical support in fixing it (or guiding them to an appropriate place to resolve the issue). The information technology office may also be aware of campus free computer programs (if they are available). Some universities have programs in which laptop computers are loaned to students who do not have the financial means to afford one.

Career Services

Most universities have a career services office that assists students with obtaining an internship or job (post-graduation). They help students with developing a resume, writing a personal statement or cover letter, and practicing interviewing skills. They also may have connections to help with job placement. Often, the career services will organize a career fair where they bring in potential employers for students to meet with on campus. Though the need for career consultation may not come about later in your teen's college, it's a helpful resource for them to have on their radar.

Resident Assistant

If your teen plans on living on campus, their resident assistant is a helpful resource. They are typically a more advanced undergraduate student (or even graduate student) who has experience being on campus. Not only are they there to help resolve any roommate difficulties (or let students into their room if they forgot or lost their keys), but they may also be able to guide them to resources on campus that may be helpful. Students should not be afraid to ask them for advice on navigating college life or where to find certain resources on campus.

Office of the Dean of Students

Hopefully this won't be the case for your teen, but should students experience any difficulties with a professor, teaching assistant, or peer that cannot be resolved and need to be reported, the Office of the Dean of Students may be a good place to start. Filing a grievance could be in response to bias or discrimination or other student misconduct. The Office of the Dean of Students may also be able to assist with support in areas such as assault and violence, grief, food or housing insecurity, assistance with catching up on work following hospitalization, or financial assistance.

Though there are many resources that can be used to assist your teen, it is often difficult to know where and how to access them. Though your teen could find these resources in the exact moment they need them, often teens feel overwhelmed when they need help. Therefore, it's helpful for your teen to have (at the very least) a vague knowledge of the places and types of support they can receive.

POST-CHAPTER ACTIVITIES

After you have become familiar with the types of university resources available to students, it is time for your teen to do the same. The post-chapter activity is designed for you and your teen to become acquainted with where and how to access the resources mentioned in this chapter at the university that they've enrolled in. With your teen, complete the "University Scavenger Hunt" to introduce you and your teen to the many supports that exist on their university campus.

Remember to mark off the completion of this chapter and the corresponding worksheets on the "Preparing for College Checklist" (see Chapter 1). Be sure to have your teen save a picture of the completed worksheets in the designated spot on their phone or computer.

University Scavenger Hunt

The number of resources available at college can feel overwhelming! The best way to access these services is often online, and this worksheet provides you with a place to hunt down and record practical contact details for the resources most helpful to *you*. Knowing where to find support can significantly enhance your college experience, ensuring you have the support you need to succeed.

Academic Resources

Academic resources provide tools and support, such as study guides and workshops, to help you excel in classes and manage your coursework.

Academic Advising	Disability Resource Center
Academic advising helps you choose your classes, plan your major, and stay on track for graduation. Email Address: _____ Phone Number: _____ Office Location: _____ Website URL: _____ Hours of Operation: _____	This center provides accommodations and services to ensure you have equal access to education and campus life. Email Address: _____ Phone Number: _____ Office Location: _____ Website URL: _____ Hours of Operation: _____
Tutoring Services	**Library Assistance**
One-on-one and group tutoring services help you understand course material and improve your grades. Email Address: _____ Phone Number: _____ Office Location: _____ Website URL: _____ Hours of Operation: _____	College librarians are invaluable resources for research, helping you navigate books, articles, and databases. Email Address: _____ Phone Number: _____ Office Location: _____ Website URL: _____ Hours of Operation: _____
Writing Center	**Office Hours**
This center supports students in all stages of their writing, from brainstorming ideas to editing their final draft. Email Address: _____ Phone Number: _____ Office Location: _____ Website URL: _____ Hours of Operation: _____	Professors and teaching assistants (TAs) often hold office hours for specific courses to help students master content. Course #1 name: _____ Office hours: _____ Course #2 name: _____ Office hours: _____ Course #3 name: _____ Office hours: _____

Physical and Mental Health Resources

Physical and mental health resources, such as mental health counseling, physical health care, and wellness programs, are offered by colleges to support your overall well-being.

Student Health Center	Counseling Center
This center provides medical services and healthcare to students, from routine check-ups to urgent care.	This center provides therapy to help you manage stress, anxiety, and other mental health challenges.
Email Address: _____ Phone Number: _____ Office Location: _____ Website URL: _____ Hours of Operation: _____	Email Address: _____ Phone Number: _____ Office Location: _____ Website URL: _____ Hours of Operation: _____
Mental Health Training Clinic	**Academic Coaching**
These clinics often offer therapy and diagnostic assessment services provided by graduate students under supervision.	Academic coaches help you develop skills like time management, organization, and study strategies.
Email Address: _____ Phone Number: _____ Office Location: _____ Website URL: _____ Hours of Operation: _____	Email Address: _____ Phone Number: _____ Office Location: _____ Website URL: _____ Hours of Operation: _____

Community Resources

Community resources help you engage with the campus community. Colleges will often host activity fairs at the beginning of each semester so students can explore their options all in one place.

Some extracurricular **student-led groups** you may consider joining include:

- ☐ Greek life (e.g., fraternities, sororities)
- ☐ Academic groups (e.g., pre-med, pre-dental, pre-law, Quiz Bowl)
- ☐ Recreational activities (e.g., intramural or club sports)
- ☐ Literature and performing arts (e.g., musical groups, acapella, bands, theater, poetry, improv)
- ☐ Cultural organizations (e.g., student-run groups for specific racial and ethnic backgrounds, LGBTQ community, religious groups, Women in STEM)
- ☐ Service-based groups (e.g., volunteering in the community)

There may also be **university-run offices or centers** for students to get involved in:

- ☐ Become a campus tour guide through the college admissions office
- ☐ Join the Reserve Officer Training Corps (ROTC)
- ☐ Join college-run cultural centers, offices, or religious spaces

GROUP: _____	GROUP: _____
Description of group:	**Description of group:**
Email Address: _____	Email Address: _____
Phone Number: _____	Phone Number: _____
Office Location: _____	Office Location: _____
Website URL: _____	Website URL: _____
Hours of Operation: _____	Hours of Operation: _____

GROUP: _____	
Description of group:	
Email Address: _____	Phone Number: _____
Office Location: _____	Website URL: _____
Hours of Operation: _____	

Logistical Resources

Logistical resources provide you with practical assistance to navigate college life smoothly and include transportation, career services, housing, and meal plans.

Career Services	Resident Assistance
This center prepares you for your future career by offering resume reviews, job search assistance, internship placements, and interview preparation.	A Resident Assistant (RA) is an upperclassman who lives in a dorm and provides guidance and organizes activities for student residents.
Email Address: _____	Email Address: _____
Phone Number: _____	Phone Number: _____
Office Location: _____	Office Location: _____
Website URL: _____	Website URL: _____
Hours of Operation: _____	Hours of Operation: _____

Office of the Dean of Students	
This office provides resources for a variety of student needs, such as filing grievances, offering crisis assistance, and providing financial assistance (e.g., food insecurity).	
Email Address: _____	
Phone Number: _____	
Office Location: _____	
Website URL: _____	
Hours of Operation: _____	

Piecing Together the Class Schedule

Chapter Outline

- Deciding on Classes
- Selecting Class Times
- Post-Chapter Activities

Your teen's academic advisor will be an invaluable resource as they put together their class schedule throughout their time in college. This is especially true their first semester, when they are likely required to register for classes with an academic advisor during university orientation. However, many academic advisors may be unaware of your teen's diagnosis of ADHD, the unique needs of students with ADHD, and the alternative planning to address these concerns. This chapter will provide class schedule considerations as well as ways in which you and your teen may advocate for them.

DECIDING ON CLASSES

Each university, college, or major may differ in the number of credits required to graduate. Further, the number of credits each course holds (e.g., 3 credits, 4 credits) varies across universities and classes, especially if there are discussion or lab sections included. Academic advisors may offer your teen a plan for them to efficiently complete their major requirements (i.e., in four years). However, depending on how demanding your teen's major is, the other responsibilities they hold (e.g., sports, working, family responsibilities), and ADHD-related difficulties, it may be difficult for your teen to complete their coursework successfully by following the "traditional" four-year plan. Therefore, you and your teen may need to advocate for taking an alternative path to best ensure their success.

Students may want to opt to take a lighter course load (e.g., four classes per semester instead of five). By doing so, your student may have to take a course or two over summers to make up for the reduction or extend their time in college (e.g., five years in college vs. four). Though your teen may not be thrilled with having to spend an extra year in college or with taking classes over the summer, it may be a practical solution if they are unable to complete all their academic tasks or their course load is creating too much stress. This could be something that your teen decides pre-emptively, by electing to take a lighter course load at the beginning of the semester. Alternatively, students may want to register for the typical load and determine mid-semester if it would be helpful to drop a course if they are struggling with the full course load. Each university will have a date by which a student can drop a course while receiving a reimbursement for the credits paid and not having any indication of doing so on their transcript. This date will be an important one to note each semester—so put it on the calendar!

Another class consideration is regarding the type of classes your teen is taking each semester. Science, Technology, Engineering, and Math (STEM) classes are often quite demanding, and it may be prudent to not take too many of these classes in any one given semester (e.g., 2–3 STEM classes, with the remaining courses being general education requirements). Not only may the material in the courses be especially challenging, but these courses often contain discussion sections or lab sections that will fill your teen's schedule and result in additional assignments. Similarly, if there are other subjects that your teen may struggle with (e.g., writing, English, foreign language), it would be wise to spread these courses across multiple semesters. In sum, your teen should avoid enrolling in all difficult or challenging classes in any given semester.

SELECTING CLASS TIMES

Let's face it: we all have times when we are more or less able to focus. It's important for your teen to acknowledge what times of the day they feel best suited to sit in classes. While some students feel most fresh and at their best in the morning, others feel afternoons are the time when they feel best able to pay attention. When possible, your teen should schedule their most difficult courses during their "prime attention times."

It also may be helpful for your teen to consider class times versus class topics for electives. It may be that your teen is willing to take a class at an undesirable time if it means the content will be more engaging than a class at a more desirable time. For example, a class that is more intriguing to your teen (i.e., it is more aligned with their interests) but first thing in the morning may still be preferable to a course with less interesting subject matter that is scheduled at a more ideal time. Understanding what factors will help your teen be most engaged in their classes, including time, will help to ensure their academic success.

Just as class times may be important, it may be helpful to understand how many classes your teen may be able to take on during any given day. If your teen is planning to enroll in five classes, it might be helpful to have two classes on Tuesday/Thursday and three classes on Monday/Wednesday/Friday. Having too many classes on any given day may seem daunting to your teen and make it difficult to maintain concentration. It may also be helpful to determine how many hours of classes your teen may be able to handle in a row before needing a break. For instance, your teen may be okay with sitting through two classes back-to-back, but no more than that before having a break. It is also important to consider the length of classes. For instance, classes that meet three days per week tend to be shorter (e.g., 50 minutes) compared to classes that meet two days a week (e.g., 75 minutes). Therefore, it may be wise for your teen to choose classes that are shorter in duration in subjects for which they find it difficult to maintain concentration.

Many universities have increased offerings for online classes. Though this may seem convenient on the surface (i.e., not having to commute or walk to class), online classes have their own challenges. If your teen is easily distracted, then online classes might be especially difficult given that they will not be in a physical classroom and they may have both home distractions as well as online distractions (e.g., other web-browsers, social media) to contend with. If online classes are the only option, your teen should identify a distraction-free environment, including limiting access to their phone or other online content. Many online courses also tend to be asynchronous in nature, which may cause further difficulties for students with ADHD. This means that there are no set class times for the course; students in an asynchronous course have to complete readings and watch pre-recorded lecture videos largely on their own time. For instance, they may be asked to watch eight lecture videos and read four chapters of text by a certain date for an exam one month in the future, but how they do so is entirely up to the student. This may be very difficult for students who struggle with time management and planning or motivation. Therefore, students with ADHD should be cautious when considering online, asynchronous classes. Should one of these classes be necessary, it is especially important to create a plan of action to complete lectures, readings, and assignments in a timely manner (see Chapters 6 and 7).

POST-CHAPTER ACTIVITIES

You and your teen should find a time to complete the "Class Schedule Builder" worksheet. This worksheet will require you and your teen to complete a few tasks. First, you and your teen should determine what the expected course load is for undergraduates. This may require you to contact an academic advisor in the department of their chosen major. From there, you and your teen should discuss whether taking a full course load is the best plan of action for your teen. You and your teen should answer the questions on the worksheet to guide class planning (e.g., times and days to schedule class). It will be important for you and your teen to map out which classes they may want to register for and how they would fit in your teen's schedule.

Remember to mark off the completion of this chapter and the corresponding worksheets on the "Preparing for College Checklist" (see Chapter 1). Be sure to have your teen save a picture of the completed worksheets in the designated spot on their phone or computer.

Class Schedule Builder

Each semester, you can use this worksheet to help you build a weekly class schedule. First, use your answers to the following questions to inform your schedule:

How many courses will you pursue this semester? _____

What times of day are you able to focus best (e.g., morning, afternoon)? _____

In one day, what is the maximum number of...

    hours you can remain focused in class? _____

    classes you can take in one day? _____

Then, fill in the table **on the next page** with the course information you will need to visualize your week. Information should include the <u>course name</u>, <u>number of course credits</u>, <u>professor name</u>, <u>building and room number</u>, <u>date and time</u> of the course, and <u>any associated lab or discussion sections</u>. For guidance, see the example class schedule builder below.

Course #1	Course #2	Course #3	Course #4	Course #5
Psychology 101 (3 credits)	*Literature 100* (3 credits)	*Music 201* (3 credits)	*Business 343* (3 credits)	
• Professor Lin • Rm. 203 in Building H • Lecture from 8:30–10:30 a.m., Friday • Lab from 5–7 p.m., Friday	• Professor Cornwall • Rm. 310 in Building C • Lecture from 11:00 a.m.—12:30 p.m., Friday	• Professor Ford • Rm. 4 in Building F • Lecture from 1:00–2:15 p.m., Tuesdays and Thursdays	• Professor Jones • Rm. 1000 in Building J • Lecture from 2:45–4:30 p.m., Tuesdays and Thursdays	

	Sunday	Monday	Tuesday	Wednesday	Thursday	Friday	Saturday
8:00							
8:30							*Psych 101 lecture*
9:00							*Psych 101 lecture*
9:30							*Psych 101 lecture*
10:00							
10:30							*Lit. 100 lecture*
11:00							*Lit. 100 lecture*
11:30							
12:00							
12:30							
1:00				*Music 201 lecture*		*Music 201 lecture*	
1:30				*Music 201 lecture*		*Music 201 lecture*	
2:00							
2:30				*Business 343 lecture*		*Business 343 lecture*	
3:00				*Business 343 lecture*		*Business 343 lecture*	

	Sunday	Monday	Tuesday	Wednesday	Thursday	Friday	Saturday
3:30							
4:00							
4:30							
5:00						*Psych 101 lecture*	
5:30							
6:00							
6:30							
7:00							
7:30							
8:00							
8:30							
9:00							

Class Schedule Builder

On the grid provided below and for each course you want to take, write down the course name, number of course credits, professor name, building and room number, date and time of the course, and any associated lab or discussion sections.

Course #1	Course #2	Course #3	Course #4	Course #5

On the weekly calendar provided below, color in time blocks relevant to each course.

	Sunday	Monday	Tuesday	Wednesday	Thursday	Friday	Saturday
8:00							
8:30							
9:00							
9:30							
10:00							
10:30							
11:00							
11:30							
12:00							
12:30							
1:00							
1:30							
2:00							

	Sunday	Monday	Tuesday	Wednesday	Thursday	Friday	Saturday
2:30							
3:00							
3:30							
4:00							
4:30							
5:00							
5:30							
6:00							
6:30							
7:00							
7:30							
8:00							
8:30							
9:00							

12

Academic Accommodations

What Are They Good For?

Chapter Outline

- Helpful Academic Accommodations
- Getting Access to Academic Accommodations
- How to Use Academic Accommodations
- Barriers to Academic Accommodations
- A Note on Learning Disorders
- Post-Chapter Activities

Academic accommodations are one important resource for many college students with ADHD. If your teen had an Individualized Education Plan (IEP) or 504 Plan in elementary, middle, or high school, academic accommodations in college operate in a similar fashion. Under the Americans with Disabilities Act (ADA) and Section 504 of the Rehabilitation Act, universities are legally required to provide academic adjustments or resources if a student has a documented physical, mental, or sensory disability. ADHD is a condition that falls within the confines of this legislation and allows students access to academic accommodations. This chapter will describe academic accommodations that are often helpful for college students with ADHD, outline the general process to acquire them through disability resource centers on your teen's campus, and help to problem-solve any barriers that your teen may experience to using them. The term "disability resource center" will be used throughout this chapter, though some universities refer to them by a different name (e.g., accessibility and disability service office, accessibility resource center).

Despite academic accommodations being one of the most common resources used by college students with ADHD, there are mixed results as to how effective they are. Academic accommodations do not teach new skills or strategies. They simply shape the academic environment to accommodate a student's disability, in this case ADHD. Therefore, though academic accommodations certainly serve a purpose (as will be described below), it is important not to view them as a cure-all. Academic accommodations may help to ensure your teen's success in college as they learn the skills outlined in Chapters 5–7 with or without professional assistance (see Chapter 13).

HELPFUL ACADEMIC ACCOMMODATIONS

There are many accommodations that are available to students on campus to ensure their academic success. The accommodation plan is individualized to address each student's difficulties inside and outside of the classroom. Though the following list of accommodations are typical ones that are frequently used to address ADHD-related difficulties in the classroom, they are by no means exhaustive of the types of accommodations that can be provided. The following accommodations are also focused on ADHD-related difficulties. If your teen has any co-occurring mental health or medical disabilities, they may be entitled to additional accommodations to ensure their college success.

Extended Time on Tests

One of the most frequently used academic accommodations among college students with ADHD is additional time on tests and quizzes. Given the attentional difficulties associated with ADHD, it may be helpful for students with ADHD to have additional time to complete timed tasks. Additional time may allow for students with ADHD to re-read instructions and questions to ensure important information isn't missed. Extended time may also grant students enough time to complete all questions given potential distractions that could impede performance. Typically, students with ADHD who receive an "extended time" accommodation will receive 1.5 to 2 times the standard allotted time to complete a test or quiz (e.g., if a test is administered during a 50-minute class period, extended time accommodations would allow a student to have 75 to 100 minutes to complete that test). A related accommodation students may access is having a designated time (e.g., 5–10 minutes) to take a break during a testing administration. This could be helpful to combat any symptoms of hyperactivity (e.g., fidgeting, restlessness) that may impede test performance.

Distraction-Reduced Testing Environment

Often used in combination with an extended testing accommodation is using an environment with reduced distractions to complete tests. The majority of the time, exams are administered in the class where the course is taught, and your teen is likely taking their exam with anywhere from 25 to 200 other students in the classroom (depending on the class enrollment). This may be incredibly distracting. Your teen may encounter other students asking questions of the professor or teaching assistant during the exam, walking to the front of the classroom to turn in their exam throughout the testing period, or opening and closing the classroom door throughout the testing period. Therefore, it could be helpful for your teen to take their exams in an environment with fewer distractions. Your teen's university likely offers more private spaces to take exams through the disability resource center. There your teen will be proctored by a staff member and will have access to a private testing room, secluded desk, or testing booth, or at the very least a room where there are fewer students completing an exam. If your teen opts to use an extended time accommodation, they typically are also required to do so in the university testing center (which is a distraction-reduced environment).

Note-Taking Resources

Campuses offer a wide variety of accommodations that facilitate note-taking and may be helpful for college students with ADHD. The first is through the receipt of a peer note-taker. Peer note-takers are coordinated through the disability resource center. Staff members will reach out to students enrolled in your teen's class and ask if there is anyone who would agree to being a peer-noter and provide their notes to a student with a disability. Your teen would remain anonymous throughout this process and notes would be shared through the disability resource center. This is helpful if your teen struggles with keeping up with taking notes during class. However, this accommodation should not be a substitute for taking notes themselves. The notes provided by classmates should only be used to supplement (or to fill in the gaps) in your teen's notes, not as a replacement.

Another note-taking accommodation that is often granted to students with ADHD is the use of a recorder to capture lecture material. If your teen becomes distracted and misses parts of a professor's lecture, the use of a recorder could provide them with the ability to go back and listen to any parts that were missed during class. Through accommodations at the disability resource center, students may also be able to request access to a professor's written notes or slides if they are not typically made available to the entire class. As stated before, this should not replace class attendance or a student's own notes, but be used as a supplement to ensure complete capturing of the class material.

Flexible Deadlines

One accommodation that is a bit of a double-edged sword is flexible deadlines. Flexible deadlines refer to a student's ability to turn in assignments after the due date without repercussions to a student's grade. However, many professors require a student to reach out and ask for an extension ahead of the due date (e.g., requesting an extension the day before an assignment is due to ask for more time vs. requesting an extension after an assignment is past due). On the one hand, this flexibility ensures that your student will not lose points or receive no credit for an assignment if they need additional time to complete it. However, it could inadvertently encourage procrastination. For example, if your teen approaches their work with the mindset of "well, I could always turn that in late," it could cause a backlog of assignments and strengthen bad habits. Extensions should be seen as a back-up option and only used occasionally when there is a legitimate reason for not being able to complete work. These extensions could be helpful while your teen works to build organization and time management skills (see Chapter 6).

Excused Absences

Similar to flexible deadlines, excused absences (or tardiness) are also both helpful and harmful as an accommodation. This accommodation would allow your child to miss class or arrive late due to their disability (i.e., ADHD). Though this could be helpful in that your teen would not be penalized for missing class or arriving late, it has its downsides as well in that this accommodation may also reinforce poor time management. Therefore, it is important to use this flexibility around attendance as a back-up plan in case an unforeseen circumstance comes up or while your teen is developing better time management skills (e.g., in working with a therapist).

GETTING ACCESS TO ACADEMIC ACCOMMODATIONS

Now that you have a brief overview of common ADHD-related accommodations, it's important to outline how your teen can obtain them. The first step in obtaining academic accommodations is to study the disability resource center website to determine your teen's university's specific requirements. Each school may require slightly different documentation. Students are typically required to complete a short background application that asks students how their disability affects their academics, past accommodations they've received (if applicable), and what types of accommodations they feel would benefit them in college. Students are also required to submit documentation of their diagnosis. This documentation can come in many forms (and may vary from school to school). A previous report from a licensed mental health professional (e.g., neuropsychological assessment, psychoeducational assessment) or a 504 or IEP plan may suffice. Other times, a university may have specific forms that they require providers to complete about a student's symptoms. The provider could be a pediatrician, psychiatrist, psychologist, social worker, or other mental health professional who can speak to your teen's symptoms and establish a formal diagnosis. If your teen does not have an established diagnosis of ADHD, it's crucial that you and your teen schedule an appointment with a mental health provider to receive a diagnosis and the accompanying documentation as soon as possible.

Once these forms are submitted, it is likely that your teen will then be asked to meet with a member of the disability resource staff. This meeting will help your teen determine what accommodations will be most beneficial for their academic success. Though these staff members will likely have recommendations for accommodations, it's important that your teen advocate for any additional accommodations that they want in their accommodation letter. Following this meeting, the disability resource center will formulate a list of accommodations that professors must abide by. Professors are not required to provide accommodations that are not on this list. Therefore, it's important that every accommodation needed is documented. Students can have an accommodation letter updated (e.g., to change or add an accommodation), but this process requires time and effort by your teen. It's best to be thoughtful and extensive when the original academic accommodation letter is created so that your teen can avoid multiple trips to this campus center.

HOW TO USE ACADEMIC ACCOMMODATIONS

The logistics of using academic accommodations may differ from university to university. Therefore, it's important for your teen to have a conversation during their initial meeting with disability resource staff on the specific steps to requesting and using their accommodations. However, there are several general guidelines that are likely to apply to any institution of higher education. Following receipt of an accommodation letter, it is the student's responsibility to notify the professor of the necessary accommodations needed. Your teen should write an email and send it to any professor (and the associated teaching assistant) with their accommodation letter attached. In that email, it is important for your teen to notify the professor of which accommodations they would like to use in the course. Though most professors do not need to meet with students to apply accommodations to the course, it may be helpful for your teen to offer to meet with them to review any questions or concerns that your teen is requesting. Below is a sample email that your teen may elect to use.

> Dear Professor Hartley,
>
> I am writing to provide you with my accommodation letter from the disability resource center. For this class, I am requesting extended time and flexible deadlines for assignments. I would be happy to meet with you to review any of these accommodations or answer any questions. Thank you for helping to ensure my success in your course.
>
> Sincerely,
> Sean

Following this email or meeting with a professor, they will grant your teen the documented accommodations and coordinate with the disability resource center should any collaboration be necessary.

In addition to contacting professors at the beginning of the semester to provide the accommodation letter, it is important that your teen stay in contact throughout the semester should they need to use any additional accommodations. It's also important to notify professors of the need for an extended deadline *before* the due date. For example, if a paper needs to be submitted by 11:59 p.m. on Sunday, it's important that your teen contact the professor before the deadline (preferably several days before the due date) rather than at 10:00 a.m. on Monday. Being proactive and discussing this need early will ensure that there are no issues with applying that accommodation.

As I mentioned at the beginning of this section, each university will have different step-by-step processes for testing accommodations. Typically students will need to log into a web-based system (or email the disability resource center) to request a space and a time to take an exam with extended time and in a private testing space. It is important to also complete this task early (e.g., one week before the test). These spaces may fill up, so booking a time early will help to avoid this problem.

BARRIERS TO ACADEMIC ACCOMMODATIONS

Occasionally students will elect not to use their accommodations, taking a reactive (vs. a proactive) approach. For example, a student may say they want to try taking a test without their accommodations for the first exam and then decide whether or not they should use them for the remaining ones. One way this could play out is that the student doesn't finish the exam or perform as well as initially expected, receives a poor grade, and then has to spend the rest of the semester trying to boost their grade. The more optimal approach would be to use the accommodations from the beginning. Students may end up finishing the exam within the standard allotted time, but they would at least have had the option for more time. Ultimately, when and how students use their accommodations is their decision, but conversations around this could be helpful in guiding them to the best decision.

Another barrier to consistently using accommodations is fear of negative evaluation from professors. Many students are afraid to approach their professor about their accommodations for fear that professors will think they are trying to game the system or get a leg up on other students. When challenging these beliefs, it's helpful to use a metaphor about running a race. As mentioned in Chapter 3, brains of emerging adults with ADHD function a bit differently. Using the racing metaphor, this would be like starting a race a half of a lap behind other runners. Accommodations don't give students a head start; they close that gap so that they are starting at the same place as other students. However, some professors may hold inappropriate beliefs about accommodations. If your teen should experience any difficulties from professors about having access to their accommodations, they should contact the disability resource center immediately for their help in intervening.

A NOTE ON LEARNING DISORDERS

This chapter has largely focused on accommodations for ADHD. However, learning disorders commonly occur with ADHD. In fact, up to 45% of children with ADHD have a co-occurring specific learning disorder (LD). Learning disorders refer to a child's difficulties in reading, writing, math, and speech and language. These difficulties in combination with ADHD symptoms may further impact academic achievement. Therefore, ensuring students with learning disorders have access to accommodations can alleviate some of the barriers for academic achievement. Though many of the academic accommodations for ADHD discussed in this chapter are also applicable, there are ones specific to LDs too. Accommodations for a reading LD may be addressed through receiving assistive technology (e.g., software that converts text to speech or speech to text). They could also include being granted audiobooks in place of (or in addition to) textbooks, to have the ability to have written material read to the student. Further, students may be able to have assistance with reading written material for exams. Difficulties with working memory may be accommodated with the ability to use memory aids like worksheets with formulas, definitions, or key terms during exams. A math LD could be accommodated with a student being allowed to use a calculator. A writing LD could be accommodated with the ability to take exams orally instead of by writing. These sorts of accommodations, specific to LDs, can help to ensure students with LDs have access to all the assistance they need to succeed academically during college. If your teen has a diagnosis of an LD, it will be important for this to be included in their application for academic accommodations. If you suspect your teen has a specific LD and would like them to be assessed, please see the "Initiating New Care" section of Chapter 13 to learn more about the process of LD diagnosis.

POST-CHAPTER ACTIVITIES

After becoming familiar with the typical accommodations for students with ADHD and the general process for obtaining accommodations, complete the "Academic Accommodations" worksheet with your teen. This will help your teen to be prepared when meeting with the disability resource center. You and your teen should also schedule an appointment with the disability resource center at your teen's university. It would be ideal to take care of this matter before arriving to campus their freshman year or at the beginning of a semester, instead of during the midst of the semester when they are juggling classes and assignments.

Remember to mark off the completion of this chapter and the corresponding worksheets on the "Preparing for College Checklist" (see Chapter 1). Be sure to have your teen save a picture of the completed worksheets in the designated spot on their phone or computer.

Accommodations Worksheet

The Americans with Disabilities Act (ADA) and Section 504 of the Rehabilitation Act legally require colleges to provide academic adjustments and resources to students with documented physical, mental, or sensory disabilities. ADHD falls within this legislation, and you can use this worksheet to help navigate accessing accommodations.

Accommodations Checklist

Mark the accommodations you think might be helpful:

- ☐ Extended time on tests (1.5–2x the allotted time)
- ☐ Designated break time on tests
- ☐ Distraction-reduced testing environment
- ☐ Note-taking resources
    - ☐ Peer note-taker
    - ☐ Recording lectures
- ☐ Flexible deadlines
- ☐ Excused absences

How to Secure Accommodations

1. **Do your research.**
   Review your college's disability resource center's website for their specific requirements for documentation.
2. **Complete background documentation.**
   Typically, students complete a short background application that describes...
   (a) how their disability affects their academics,
   (b) any past accommodations received, if applicable, and
   (c) types of accommodations you might benefit from in in college.
3. **Complete diagnosis documentation.**
   In addition, you will provide documentation of your diagnosis (e.g., neuropsychological assessment, 504/IEP plan). If documentation is unavailable, the college will provide you with a form for a healthcare provider to complete.
4. **Formulate the accommodations letter.**
   With disability resource center staff, you will discuss which accommodations might be most beneficial and finalize your accommodations letter.
5. **Share your letter with professors.**
6. **Update accommodations.**
   Accommodation letters can be updated any time by contacting the disability resource center.

Your Disability Resource Center

Name: _____
Address: _____
Phone Number: _____
E-mail: _____

PART V

Mental Health

13

Initiating or Maintaining Mental Health Care

Chapter Outline

- Maintaining Pharmacological Care
- Maintaining Psychosocial Therapeutic Care
- Initiating New Care
- Medication Use, Diversion, and Safe Storage
- Post-Chapter Activities

The transition to college brings about many changes including potential shifts in your teen's healthcare. As you and your teen prepare for this developmental stage, it is important to understand if and how your teen is going to maintain their current care or if new care needs to be initiated. This information is also applicable if your teen should decide to pursue any mental health care in the future.

MAINTAINING PHARMACOLOGICAL CARE

It's possible that your teen may be currently prescribed medications for ADHD or for other mental health conditions (e.g., depression, anxiety). There are a variety of avenues in which families receive pharmacological care, but most commonly it is through pediatricians or psychiatrists. Therefore, prior to your child beginning their college career, it's important to discuss continued care with your providers. Typically pediatricians are willing to continue seeing their patients through the college years, though this is not a guarantee. Therefore, it's important to ensure that if your child is receiving necessary medications for their mental health through a pediatrician, that they agree to this continued care after your teen has turned 18 years old.

However, in addition to "aging out" of a pediatrician's office, there is also the concern of a pediatrician or psychiatrist being able to prescribe across state lines. This may not be a concern if your teen is attending a school within their home state. If your child is staying local, they may not need to change anything about how they receive their prescription. If they are staying within the state but not within a short distance of their regular pharmacy, it may involve you and your teen updating the provider as to what new pharmacy they want their prescriptions sent to.

Given that prescriptions to treat ADHD are most often classified as a controlled substance, if your teen is leaving the state for college there may be logistic challenges that could affect your child's ability to have continued access to their prescription medications. Your teen's pediatrician or psychiatrist may have prescription rights (i.e., they are licensed) in both your home state and the state your teen in which your teen will be attending college, but this is not common. You and your teen may need to problem solve how they will have access to their medication regularly. For instance, if they receive their medication in three-month refills, they may be able to return home during breaks to obtain the next three months' worth of medications before they run out. Not all medications are given in such large quantities (especially controlled substances), and your teen may only be able to receive a 30-day refill. If this is the case for your teen, returning to their home state each month may not be practical depending on where they are attending school.

Some pharmacies may be willing to fill a prescription across state lines. However, this depends on the pharmacy or your teen's provider. It also depends on the laws of your state. What complicates things further is that each state has not only different laws within the state but also different guidelines with how they interact with other states. That being said, it's important to have these discussions with your teen's provider to be sure there is a reliable plan in place to ensure continuity of their medication. What you and your teen will want to avoid is scrambling to find answers to these questions when there are only seven days (or less) left in their prescription. Having these conversations early is key to ensuring a smooth transition. If your provider indicates that you will need to find alternative care, the section "Initiating New Care" in this chapter will help to guide you through that process.

MAINTAINING PSYCHOSOCIAL THERAPEUTIC CARE

In addition to receiving necessary medications, continuing with a psychosocial therapy provider (e.g., psychologist, social worker, counselor) may be subject to your child's age and physical location. If your child's mental health care provider is located within a pediatric unit, there is a chance they will no longer qualify for services there, though this is rare. However, it is important to check on this early so that you and your teen have ample time to find a new provider if necessary.

If your child is staying local for college and there are no age restrictions, there should not be any cause for looking for alternative care. If your child is staying within state but too far to have in-person sessions with a mental health provider, it is important that you and your teen check with their current provider that they offer telehealth sessions (i.e., sessions over a secure video conferencing platform like Zoom). Since the pandemic, many therapists have shifted to a hybrid approach where they allow patients to be seen in person or over the internet. Determining that this is the case with your child's provider will be important to ensuring continued care when your teen transitions to college.

If your child is moving out of state for college, there is a greater likelihood that your teen may need to find a new mental health provider. Some therapists hold licenses to practice in multiple states. This is especially common for therapists who are close to the border of other states (e.g., a therapist in New York City may have licenses in New Jersey and Connecticut; a therapist in Washington DC may have licenses in Virginia and Maryland). In addition to therapists holding multiple licenses, the PSYPACT organization was created to help with therapists being able to provide telepsychology sessions across state lines. However, even if your therapist is a member of PSYPACT, not all states have approved cross-state practice through this legislation. You can learn more about what states have approved PSYPACT at their website: https://psypact.org/. Be sure to ask your teen's therapist about this possibility.

Many teens prefer to have in-person sessions or find them more productive and with less distractions. Therefore, even if your teen's mental health provider does offer telehealth sessions, it's important to discuss with your teen what they feel would be most helpful during this transition: continuity (i.e., having the same provider but meeting over the internet) or in-person sessions (i.e., having in-person sessions but with a new provider). If their decision involves finding a new provider, reading the following section will be important.

INITIATING NEW CARE

Whether your teen is switching to a new provider or wanting to initiate care for the first time, there are several avenues that may be beneficial in locating a new provider (whether it be for prescriptions or therapy sessions). The first place to start is with their current provider, if your teen has one. They may have colleagues in other states they could refer your teen to or networks they can contact on your teen's behalf. If your child does not have a current provider or their current provider has no referrals, you may choose to contact the counseling center of the university they plan to attend. They may have referrals that they provide to students to access care in the community. If your current provider or the college counseling center do not have suggestions, you may need to reach out independently to find care. Following is a list of organizations that might be helpful in finding a mental health provider.

In searching independently for a provider, you could consider browsing the Children and Adults with ADHD (CHADD) website, which is a resource for individuals with ADHD (https://chadd.org/affiliate-locator). There are professional sites like the American Psychological Association (locator.apa.org) and the Association for Behavioral and Cognitive Therapies (abct.org), where you may find a psychologist in your teen's new area. For psychiatrists, you could try organizations like the American Psychiatric Association (https://finder.psychiatry.org/s/). Members of these organizations are professionals in the field and opt to provide information as to whether they see patients. These websites are also great resources for finding evidence-based care. Similarly, the site PsychologyToday (psychologytoday.com) serves as a platform for mental health professionals to advertise their services and indicate their expertise. On this site you may want to search for providers with expertise in ADHD, cognitive-behavioral therapy, or organizational skills and time management. You can also filter results based on aspects such as location, demographic factors of the therapist, the type of degree the therapist holds, and the type of insurance the therapist accepts. You can also search for psychiatrists on this site. You may also opt to search for a therapist through your insurance company's website.

In addition to identifying a new provider for your teen that has expertise in evidence-based treatments for ADHD (e.g., cognitive-behavioral therapy, or organizational skills and time management), you may want to inquire about the use of specific manuals for ADHD treatment. A few examples are *Cognitive-Behavioral Therapy for Adult ADHD*; *Mastering Your Adult ADHD*; *Thriving in College with ADHD*; and *CBT for College Students with ADHD*. These manuals have been developed by experts in the field to guide therapists in treating young adults with ADHD. The full information for these titles is in the bibliography.

As first mentioned in Chapter 12, many college students with ADHD have a co-occurring learning disorder. Though many will have already received formal testing and a diagnosis, it is never too late for testing if you or your teen suspect a learning disorder. If interested, you should search for a local psychologist who can provide psychoeducational assessment in your area. Unfortunately, insurance companies' coverage of psychoeducational assessment is limited. Therefore, it would be ideal to have this testing done for free through your teen's public school system (if applicable). The earlier you pursue this option the better as there could be a waiting list to receive psychoeducational testing. Other affordable options may be through university training clinics which often offer this service on a sliding scale. You may want to consider searching for psychoeducational assessment at universities located near your area or near the university your teen will enroll in. This psychoeducational testing may be offered for free through your teen's university. I recommend contacting the disability resource center or counseling center at their university to inquire about whether psychoeducational testing is provided through the university or if they have local recommendations.

MEDICATION USE, DIVERSION, AND SAFE STORAGE

Many students with ADHD will continue taking or wish to begin taking prescription medication for ADHD during their years in college. The following sections will describe ways in which your teen can continue to adhere to their medication routine, initiate new pharmacological care, and store medication safely.

Medication Use During College

Throughout their childhood and adolescence, as a parent, you've likely played a major role in ensuring that your teen is taking any prescription medications. As high schoolers transition to college, it's developmentally appropriate for them to take responsibility for taking their medications. However, the forgetfulness associated with ADHD may make it difficult for them to assume this task independently without any support. It could be helpful to discuss ways to support them in taking on this responsibility.

The best way you can support your teen in assuming responsibility for their medication regimen is by helping them list ideas for better remembering to take their medications. You should do so using the communication skills discussed in Chapter 2. After listing ideas, you may want to supplement your teen's solutions with the following (if they don't come up with these solutions themselves). Students may want to use a daily reminder or alarm on their cell phone to alert them to take their medication. This will help students not only take their medication daily, but at the same time each day. They may also want to consider using a daily medication dose holder to store a week's worth of medication and be able to verify that they took their medication. Students also may want to store this medication holder in a visible location so that they know where their medication is and so its presence can serve as a reminder.

Your teen may want or need check-ins with you as to whether they remembered to take their medication. Some teens may find this overbearing. Others may find this supportive. Therefore, discussing what would be helpful is a must. This level of checking in also may change over time. It would be most helpful for you to begin transferring this responsibility to your teen before they leave for college, allow them time to practice with your support, and assume responsibility when they leave for school.

Medication Diversion and Safe Storage

If your teen is prescribed stimulant medication (or any other controlled substances), it's important to discuss safely storing their medications and not sharing medications with peers. Diversion refers to an individual sharing or selling their prescription medication. Stimulant diversion among college students is common, with up to 30% of college students with ADHD reporting having given, sold, or traded their medications with someone else. With students gaining greater independence during their transition to college and potentially living away from home, it's important to discuss the consequences of diversion and how to store medication safely.

Any stimulant diversion may have severe ramifications. Your teen may not think much of sharing one pill with a friend who asks. However, one act is enough for negative consequences, and if word spreads that your teen has shared their prescription stimulants, they might be approached by more peers, which increases the likelihood that resident assistants, school officials, or anyone in a position of authority learns of this illegal activity. This illicit behavior could result in academic consequences (e.g., suspension, expulsion) or even legal action against your teen.

Though raising these negative consequences with your teen could be helpful in reducing the risk of diversion, it may be more effective coming from their prescribing physician or psychiatrist. Before your teen begins college, it may be worthwhile to ask their prescriber (or therapist) to provide information and discuss the consequences of stimulant diversion. Following that conversation, you may want to reinforce this information. Unfortunately, there is also a risk of students' medication being stolen while away at college, so it could also be helpful to discuss where your teen will store their medication. They may want to have a weekly dose container for their medication but store the rest in a more hidden location (e.g., in a clothing drawer or locked box). This could help medication from being taken by a roommate or fellow student living in the dorms.

It's important to initiate conversations with current or new providers early. Therapists often have waitlists, or it may take time for your teen to schedule an assessment and be enrolled in services. Therefore, as soon as your child determines where they will be enrolling, you and your teen should begin conversations with current or prospective providers. It also may be that you and your teen decide that pharmacological or therapeutic care is not needed at the beginning of college. However, should that change, knowing the steps to find a reliable provider helps to expedite the process from searching to enrollment.

POST-CHAPTER ACTIVITIES

In preparation for maintaining or initiating mental health care, please review and complete the "Mental Health Care" worksheet with your teen to determine their plan for their mental health care. The answers to your questions may result in the need to talk with existing or new providers. Additionally, you may wish to ask your teen's medication prescriber (if they have one) to have a discussion with your teen about medication diversion.

Remember to mark off the completion of this chapter and the corresponding worksheets on the "Preparing for College Checklist" (see Chapter 1). Be sure to have your teen save a picture of the completed worksheets in the designated spot on their phone or computer.

Mental Health Care

Your transition to college may bring about big changes in how you approach your mental health care. Use this worksheet to identify your current healthcare needs, as well as how to continue or establish care with mental health providers (e.g., therapists, counselors) and medical providers (e.g., psychiatrists, family doctors) while in college.

Managing Therapeutic Care

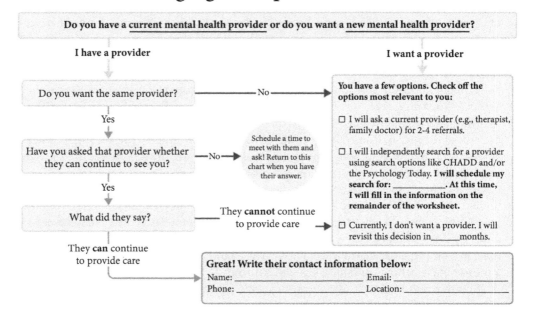

When looking for a mental health provider, ask yourself the following:

What would you like to work on with your provider (e.g., time management, emotion regulation)? _____
_____
_____

How often would you like to meet (e.g., once a week, twice a month)? _____

> **Cognitive Behavioral Therapy** (CBT) and **Organizational Skills Training** (OST) are evidence-based treatments shown to be effective for mananging ADHD symptoms. CBT helps individuals develop strategies to change negative thought patterns and behaviors, while OST focuses on improving time management, planning, and organizational skills. When seeking a new provider, consider those who utilize specific treatment manuals such as *Cognitive Behavioral Therapy for Adult ADHD* by Solanto (2011), *Mastering Your Adult ADHD: A Cognitive-Behavioral Treatment Progam, Therapists Guide* by Safren, Sprich, Perlman, & Otto (2017), and *Thriving in College with ADHD* by Canu, Knouse, Flory, & Hartung (2023).

List mental health providers you intend to contact:
Name and Email/Phone: _____
Name and Email/Phone: _____
Name and Email/Phone: _____

Managing Pharmacological Care

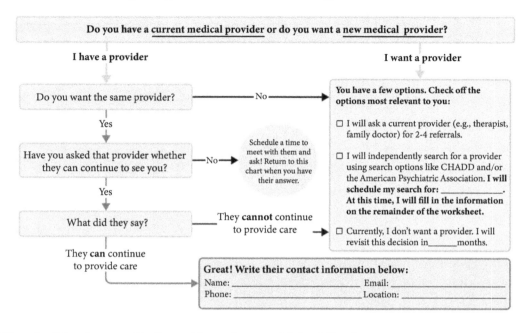

When looking for a medical provider, ask yourself the following:

What do you hope to feel/experience when using medication for ADHD (e.g., more focus, less overwhelm)?
_____
_____
_____

What side effects might you want to mention to your provider if they arise (e.g., poor appetite, irritability)?
_____
_____

How might you react if someone asks to use your medication?
_____
_____

When would you prefer to take your medications (e.g., morning, night)?
_____

How will you remember to take your medications (e.g., timers, a pill box)?
_____

List medical providers you intend to contact:
Name and Email/Phone: _____
Name and Email/Phone: _____
Name and Email/Phone: _____
Name and Email/Phone: _____
Name and Email/Phone: _____

14

Dealing with Depression

Chapter Overview

- What is Depression?
- Depression and ADHD
- Addressing Negative Mood
- Addressing Parental Depression
- Post-Chapter Activities

Depression is one mental health condition that frequently co-occurs with ADHD, and is especially prevalent during the college years. The chapter will discuss what depression is, how your teen can monitor mood, and what your teen should do if they face depression. It will also present information about how you can ease potential feelings of depression that you might encounter during your teen's transition. You may be tempted to skip this chapter if your teen is not currently experiencing any symptoms of depression, but it's much better to be informed and have an action plan before depression emerges than be trying to figure out solutions during a crisis. Therefore, it's recommended that regardless of any current mood difficulties, you learn about depression and ways to prevent or address it.

WHAT IS DEPRESSION?

Depression is a serious mental health condition that can affect everyone, regardless of gender, from childhood to late adulthood. Depression also looks different from person to person given the many symptoms associated with it. Depression can manifest as sadness or depressed mood, or as irritability and anger. Individuals experiencing depression may experience a loss of interest in the things that they typically enjoy. It can be associated with changes in sleep (too much or too little), changes in appetite (weight loss, decreased appetite or weight gain, increased appetite), and changes in motor movements (e.g., walking and talking much slower than normal or being fidgety or restless). People suffering from depression may experience loss of energy and fatigue, or have difficulty making decisions or concentrating more than normal. Depression may also result in feelings of worthlessness or suicidal thoughts and behaviors. Individuals experiencing depression don't need to experience all of these symptoms, which is why depression can look so different from person to person.

You may be wondering, "How do feelings of sadness or grief differ from a diagnosis of depression?" For a diagnosis of depression, symptoms must be present for at least two weeks and for most of the day, nearly every day during that two-week span. In other words, these symptoms must persist for an extended period of time and be present most of the time. Symptoms also must be impacting functioning at work, home, and school. Almost everybody experiences times in their life when they may be feeling down or sad—after a breakup, getting fired from a job, or getting into an argument with a friend or family member. Experiencing sadness after these events or just feeling occasionally sad in general is completely normal. It only rises to the level of a diagnosed condition when these symptoms last a considerable period of time, last most of the day (not just brief periods throughout the day), and impact a person's ability to live their life. This is not to say that subclinical depression (i.e., when symptoms are present but don't rise to the level of a diagnosable condition) is something to ignore. The later sections in this chapter will talk about when and how to address both severe and subclinical depression. Now that you have a brief overview of depression, it's important to understand how it ties in with ADHD.

DEPRESSION AND ADHD

Decades of research have indicated that college students with ADHD are at a greater risk for developing depression than their peers without ADHD; approximately 32% of college students with ADHD have a current, co-occurring depressive disorder, compared to only 5% of students without ADHD. This rate is even higher if past episodes of depression are considered. In addition to the increased odds for experiencing depression, college students with ADHD are more likely to experience more severe and recurrent episodes of depression as well as greater levels of overall impairment. Given these startling facts, it's important to understand how and why college students with ADHD may be at higher risk for depression. Work in this area has suggested that depression seen in ADHD could be the byproduct of social and academic difficulties, and biological or neurological factors.

Some researchers suggest that depression is the result of the difficulties that people with ADHD may face in social and academic areas. For instance, college students with ADHD are more likely to experience academic difficulties (e.g., forgetting to turn in assignments, receiving poor grades, failing classes) and social difficulties (e.g., conflicts with peers, difficulties forming and maintaining friendships). It may be that the result of experiencing these negative academic and social experiences is falling into depression. This would suggest that addressing these concerns alone would decrease the risk for depression.

However, studies have shown that even after accounting for academic and social difficulties, individuals with ADHD are still at a higher risk for depression. This would suggest that there may be other biological and neurological factors in play. For example, individuals with ADHD may have a less-sensitive reward system in that they do not experience the same level of positive emotion or reward as their peers without ADHD. Other research indicates that difficulties with emotion regulation might explain the link between ADHD and depression. More specifically, research has shown that individuals with ADHD have greater fluctuations in negative mood as well as more difficulty controlling or coping with negative emotions.

You may be wondering why you need to know about these underlying reasons for the link between ADHD and depression. The reason is that there may be things that your teen can do both on their own or in working with a mental health professional to prevent or treat depression.

ADDRESSING NEGATIVE MOOD

If your teen is suffering from chronic or heightened depression, the best course of action is to seek help with a mental health professional (e.g., psychologist, licensed clinical social worker). Therapists who specialize in cognitive-behavioral therapy, interpersonal therapy, or acceptance and commitment therapy may be promising avenues for treatment. In cognitive-behavioral therapy, therapists work with patients to identify negative thoughts (e.g., "I'm a terrible student," "nobody likes me") and develop more positive patterns of thinking. Therapists also help patients to increase the number of positive and productive activities in their daily life and recognize how their mood is tied to the activities that make up their day. In interpersonal therapy for depression, therapists work with patients to identify symptoms and how they affect their interpersonal relationships. In acceptance and commitment therapy, therapists help patients identify their negative emotions and rather than avoid them, approach them and not allow them to hinder moving forward with their lives. In addition to psychosocial therapies, there are medication therapies that are used to treat mood disorders. You and your teen should consult their primary care provider, or a psychiatrist should this be a treatment you wish to pursue. Alternatively, you could use the methods described in Chapter 13 for initiating new care to find a provider that best meets your teen's needs.

Should your teen be suffering from mild or occasional symptoms of depression, irritability, or homesickness, there may be some tips and tricks that could help boost their mood. Given that academic and social difficulties increase feelings of sadness in people with ADHD, improving academic performance and increasing social activities with friends could help boost mood. Completing assignments or getting help with classwork could help to increase self-esteem regarding their academic abilities. When you feel down or depressed, you might experience a downward spiral. This is demonstrated in the corresponding figure. Feelings of sadness could lead one to withdraw from things they used to enjoy. In turn, this withdrawal may cause more feelings of isolation and sadness. Breaking this downward spiral helps to alleviate feelings of sadness; forcing oneself to engage in a pleasurable activity may decrease feelings of sadness. Feeling less sad may then encourage one to continue being more active.

REVERSE THE SPIRAL

The "downward spiral" and "upward spiral" below represent how your mood and actions affect each other. In the downward spiral, feeling low makes you do less, which worsens your mood, leading you to do even less, and creating a negative cycle. On the other hand, the upward spiral starts with doing something small that makes you feel a bit better. Feeling better encourages you to do more, which further improves your mood, creating a positive cycle. What we do often precedes how we feel. This shows how taking small positive actions—even when we don't feel particularly motivated to—can help break the cycle of feeling down and improve your overall mood and activity levels.

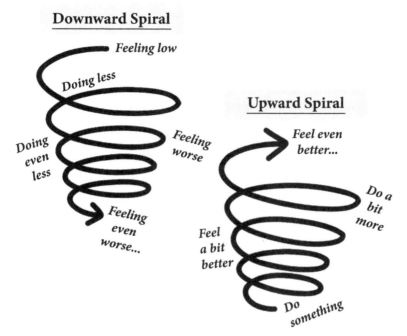

If your teen is feeling down or sad, helping them break the downward spiral and get on track with an upward one is a great solution. To make it easiest, it's helpful for your teen to have an inventory of different activities that they could engage in regardless of the time, location, and so on. This list could include things like spending time with friends or family, doing pleasant activities, or exercising to help boost mood (see post-chapter activity). Even if your teen is not currently experiencing sadness or depression, it is helpful to have a contingency plan for if (or when) these symptoms arise.

ADDRESSING PARENTAL DEPRESSION

When discussing depression, it's important to not ignore the potential for parental depression, as well. The transition to college for many parents also marks the beginning of "empty nesting" or no longer having children living at home. This can be quite a day-to-day shift for many parents, and the change may result in parents feeling uncertain about their identity and the appearance of the loss of their parental role. Ultimately, this could result in possible feelings of depression.

Parental depression has several implications for teen functioning. Not only is the tendency for depression genetic, but it can also affect the way in which caregivers parent. For example, depressive symptoms in caregivers predict adolescents' perceptions of negative parent–adolescent relationships and predict adolescents' level of perceived stress. Further, parent depression is linked with lower levels of perceived support among adolescents. This is especially important given that parental support is associated with psychological adjustment and depression among college students. To be present with and supportive of your teen, it's important to be aware of your own mental health.

POST-CHAPTER ACTIVITIES

Given the impact depression can have both on you and your teen's lives, it's important to have a plan in place for both you and your teen. In the post-chapter activity, you and your teen should complete the "Coping With Depression" worksheets together to develop a plan in case any feelings of depression arise. This activity also serves as a way for you and your teen to normalize talking about mental health concerns like depression.

Remember to mark off the completion of this chapter and the corresponding worksheets on the "Preparing for College Checklist" (see Chapter 1). Be sure to have your teen save a picture of the completed worksheets in the designated spot on their phone or computer.

Coping With Depression

Feeling sad is a normal part of life, especially when dealing with disappointments or challenges. However, depression is more than just sadness, and having ADHD puts you at higher risk for developing it. Symptoms may include the following for most of the day, almost every day, for at least two weeks:

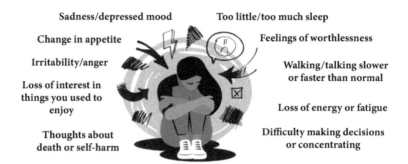

- Sadness/depressed mood
- Change in appetite
- Irritability/anger
- Loss of interest in things you used to enjoy
- Thoughts about death or self-harm
- Too little/too much sleep
- Feelings of worthlessness
- Walking/talking slower or faster than normal
- Loss of energy or fatigue
- Difficulty making decisions or concentrating

Identifying the signs of depression is crucial to seeking the right support, and it's best to catch these signs as early as possible. **Use the space below to identify what depression looks like for you:**

What do you notice yourself doing or *not* doing when feeling low? _____

What symptoms do you experience? _____

What events seem to trigger depression? _____

Now that you've recognized when you're feeling low, there are several strategies you can use to lift your mood. Think about what things and people make you feel lighter, more capable, and more fulfilled, even if you only feel that way for a moment.

Coping Strategies: Activities you can do to take your mind off of scary thoughts or sad feelings.

1. _____   4. _____
2. _____   5. _____
3. _____   6. _____

Helpful People: Reach out to people you feel safe with for support when you're feeling down.

1. Name and phone #: _____
2. Name and phone #: _____
3. Name and phone #: _____

Helpful Resources: Keep a list of important contacts for when you need extra support.

1. Therapist name and phone #: _____
2. Doctor's name and phone #: _____
3. College Counseling Center phone #: _____
4. College Crisis Phone #: _____ Suicide Hotline #: **988**

Coping With Depression as a Parent

Your child going off to college is an incredible transition—both for your child and for you. The sudden absence of a child can cause parents to question their identity, and the ensuing uncertainty can result in feelings of depression. Symptoms may include the following for most of the day, almost every day, for at least two weeks:

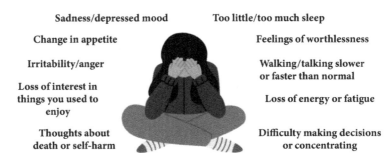

- Sadness/depressed mood
- Change in appetite
- Irritability/anger
- Loss of interest in things you used to enjoy
- Thoughts about death or self-harm
- Too little/too much sleep
- Feelings of worthlessness
- Walking/talking slower or faster than normal
- Loss of energy or fatigue
- Difficulty making decisions or concentrating

Identifying the signs of depression is crucial to seeking the right support, and it's best to catch these signs as early as possible. **Use the space below to identify what depression looks like for you:**

What do you notice yourself doing or *not* doing when feeling low? _____

What symptoms do you experience? _____

What events seem to trigger depression? _____

Now that you've recognized when you're feeling low, there are several strategies you can use to lift your mood. Think about what things and people make you feel lighter, more capable, and more fulfilled, even if you only feel that way for a moment.

Coping Strategies: Activities you can do to take your mind off of distressing thoughts or sad feelings.

1. _____ 4. _____
2. _____ 5. _____
3. _____ 6. _____

Helpful People: Reach out to people you feel safe with for support when you're feeling down.

  1. Name and phone #: _____
  2. Name and phone #: _____
  3. Name and phone #: _____

Helpful Resources: Keep a list of important contacts for when you need extra support.

  1. Therapist name and phone #: _____
  2. Doctor's name and phone #: _____
  3. Suicide Hotline #: **988**

Addressing Anxiety

Chapter Overview

- What is Anxiety?
- Anxiety and ADHD
- Addressing Anxiety
- Parental Anxiety During the Transition to College
- Post-Chapter Activities

Like depression, anxiety is another mental health condition that frequently co-occurs with ADHD. This chapter will discuss what anxiety is, why it might co-occur with ADHD, and what students should do if they experience anxiety. Like the previous chapter, it will also discuss how parental anxiety may arise as teens transition from high school to college. You and your teen may not currently be experiencing anxiety, but it's likely that at some point one or both of you will feel stressed or overwhelmed during the college years. This chapter is designed to help parents and teens learn the signs and symptoms of anxiety and know how to address them should they arise.

WHAT IS ANXIETY?

Anxiety refers to having stress, fear, or worries about one or more areas of life. Like depression, anxiety can be expressed in someone's thoughts, feelings, and behaviors. Everyone experiences anxiety from time to time—preparing to take a test, giving a speech, going on a first date. However, anxiety becomes problematic when those anxious thoughts, feelings, and behaviors begin to happen frequently and start to impact someone's daily life (i.e., their schoolwork, job, or relationships). For some, anxious thoughts begin to take over one's thinking—"If I answer the question wrong, the class will think I'm stupid"; "If I don't pass this test, I'm going to fail the class"—and it's hard to concentrate on anything else. Some people may feel physical symptoms of anxiety like headaches, stomach aches, restlessness, and quicker breathing or heartrate. Anxiety can also impact one's behaviors. Being worried may cause someone to avoid the things they're afraid of. For example, if someone is afraid of social situations, they may avoid going to parties. If someone is afraid of embarrassing themselves, they may not answer questions or talk in class. If someone is afraid of not being able to complete a homework assignment, they may avoid starting it. Successful treatments for anxiety target the thoughts, feelings, and behaviors associated with anxiety. Now that you have a brief overview of anxiety, it's important to understand it's relation with ADHD.

ANXIETY AND ADHD

Students with ADHD are at heightened risk for experiencing an anxiety disorder; 29% of college students with ADHD also have a co-occurring anxiety disorder, compared to only 3.6% of their peers without ADHD. Several explanations have been raised for why those with ADHD may be more likely to experience anxiety, including genetic predisposition, cognitive processing difficulties, struggles with executive functioning, and high levels of procrastination.

Anxiety disorders tend to run in families; individuals who have an immediate family member (e.g., parent, sibling) with an anxiety disorder are four to six times more likely to also experience anxiety, compared to those without a first-degree relative with an anxiety disorder. This may be due to specific genes related to anxiety that are passed down from parent to child. However, just because an individual may have an increased risk for anxiety due to genetics and family history doesn't mean someone is destined to experience an anxiety disorder. There are other risk or protective factors at play (which may be especially salient for individuals with ADHD). I offer some explanations below.

Some students with ADHD struggle with cognitive processing, in that they may process information slower than their peers without ADHD. This delay in processing could result in academic or social impairment and subsequently lead to anxiety. Similarly, from an executive functioning standpoint, students may have difficulty inhibiting impulses (e.g., interrupting) or making rash decisions. Difficulties with inhibition may lead to difficulties in adult life (e.g., social relationships, academics, work). As was mentioned in Chapter 3, many college students, especially those with ADHD, struggle with procrastination. Students with ADHD may put off working on a large assignment or studying for an exam—and when the deadline is only a day (or hours) away, students with ADHD experience a great deal of anxiety. In some cases this anxiety may be paralyzing, to the extent that a student may be so overcome by anxiety that they avoid doing the work altogether. By avoiding the work their anxiety decreases, but their schoolwork and grades become collateral damage.

In some cases, students report that their anxiety is motivating. For example, knowing that they are not able to procrastinate any longer due to an approaching deadline, their subsequent anxiety prompts them to complete the work. However, the degree of anxiety likely impacts whether your teen will feel motivated or not. A small amount of anxiety or pressure may encourage your teen to get their work done, but too much anxiety may be debilitating and cause your teen to shut down. Therefore, the best course of action is for your teen to learn to complete their work without having to rely on a looming deadline (and the anxiety that accompanies it) for motivation. The previous chapters on time management and organization (see Chapters 5, 6, and 7), as well as working with a professional on ADHD-related difficulties (see Chapter 13), may help your teen to preemptively avoid anxiety. The following section in this chapter will provide you and your teen with tips should your teen experience occasional bouts of stress or anxiety.

ADDRESSING ANXIETY

If your teen is experiencing clinical (or high) levels of anxiety, the best course of action is to seek help from a professional mental health provider. Mental health providers who specialize in cognitive-behavioral therapy (CBT) may be most beneficial. In CBT for anxiety, mental health providers help patients challenge anxious thoughts (e.g., "if this assignment isn't perfect, it's not worth turning in"; "I'll never be able to get this work done") and learn strategies to cope with anxiety should it arise. Therapists might also introduce components of exposure therapy, in which patients (with support from their therapist) are exposed to the situations that they find anxiety-provoking and use strategies to cope with that anxiety in the moment. These exposures help to prove to patients that they can face their fears without negative consequences.

There is no substitute for seeking professional mental health care, but if your teen is only occasionally experiencing anxiety the following tips could be helpful. First, avoidance is what often maintains anxiety. The more you are able to encourage your teen to face what is giving them anxiety or causing stress, the better off they will be. If your teen feels a task is insurmountable (e.g., a large term paper, an exam covering a lot of material), it may be helpful for you to assist them with identifying a small first step for them to accomplish and move on from there. For example, having the goal of writing one paragraph may seem more feasible than writing an entire term paper. When a task seems impossible to complete, students may have less motivation and believe they are incapable of completing it. Once your teen finishes that first, manageable goal (e.g., writing one paragraph), they should set a new goal. Getting started and completing one task helps students stay motivated to keep working.

Parents should also encourage their teens to try deep breathing or practice mindful meditation. Often anxiety manifests as rapid breathing, heartrate, or restlessness. To counter that, you should encourage your teen to try using deep breathing (i.e., taking slow deep breaths in from the diaphragm and consciously and slowly exhaling). This helps to slow breathing and heart rate. Mindfulness-based interventions have also been shown to be effective for college students. In mindfulness-based interventions, individuals train their minds to pay greater attention to physical sensations and life events. During mindfulness exercises one is asked to focus on their posture and breathing, and when the mind wanders to bring their thoughts back to breathing and posture. This helps ground the individual and alleviates the physical sensations of anxiety and anxious thoughts floating around in their head. Mindfulness exercises are often completed with a mental health provider, but they can also be completed independently. Guided meditations are available on streaming services (e.g., YouTube, Spotify, Apple Music) as well as apps specifically designed for mindfulness (e.g., Headspace, Calm).

As mentioned in the previous sections on depression, it's helpful for teens to have a series of activities that could help in coping with negative thoughts and feelings. If your teen is feeling anxious or stressed, doing an enjoyable activity—for a brief period—could be helpful. Listening to music, exercising, talking with friends, or drawing are all activities that could help combat worries. However, it's important that these activities don't become distractors. As mentioned earlier, when one is worried about or scared of something they may want to avoid it, so it's important that these coping activities don't become a permanent distraction. Setting a limit as to how long they may engage in one of these coping activities can be beneficial, so that the coping doesn't become an avoidance tactic.

PARENTAL ANXIETY DURING THE TRANSITION TO COLLEGE

In addition to students facing anxiety during the transition to college or throughout their college years, parents may also experience anxiety during this developmental period. Throughout high school you've been able to keep close tabs on your teen's progress in school; your teen showing up to school and attending class may have been assumptions that didn't require follow-up. You've likely been able to ask your teen what homework they have and if they've completed it. You've also had access to your teen's teachers and the school administration, either through email or scheduling a meeting in person. These things are likely to change as your teen transitions to college. With less face time and communication, you may be wondering or worrying about what is going on while they are away. Because of the Family Educational Rights and Privacy Act (FERPA), it is illegal for schools to share academic information with parents of students without their consent, so reassurance from teachers or schools may no longer be possible. Given these major changes, it's not uncommon that parents experience anxiety during this transition. Therefore, you may also want to consider the tools that were mentioned in the previous section if you find yourself experiencing anxiety.

POST-CHAPTER ACTIVITIES

Like the post-chapter activity you completed with your teen in Chapter 14 on depression, you and your teen should use the "Coping With Anxiety" worksheets to discuss your unique signs and symptoms of anxiety and develop a plan for what to do it if you experience stress or anxiety. This discussion is also designed to further emphasize open communication between you and your teen about any mental health concerns.

Remember to mark off the completion of this chapter and the corresponding worksheets on the "Preparing for College Checklist" (see Chapter 1). Be sure to have your teen save a picture of the completed worksheets in the designated spot on their phone or computer.

Coping With Anxiety

Feeling anxious is a normal and even essential experience—in many ways, some anxiety is helpful. However, too much anxiety can be paralyzing. Anxiety becomes problematic when anxious thoughts, feelings, and behaviors occur most of the day, nearly every day, and negatively impact your life. It commonly co-occurs with ADHD, and symptoms to look out for include:

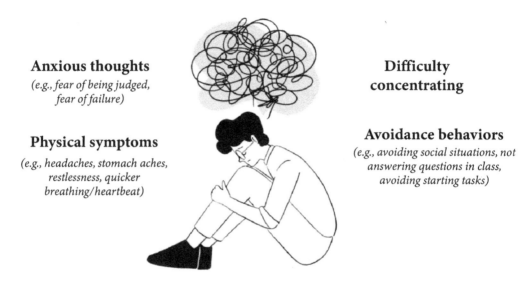

Anxious thoughts
(e.g., fear of being judged, fear of failure)

Physical symptoms
(e.g., headaches, stomach aches, restlessness, quicker breathing/heartbeat)

Difficulty concentrating

Avoidance behaviors
(e.g., avoiding social situations, not answering questions in class, avoiding starting tasks)

Identifying the signs of anxiety is crucial to seeking the right support, and it's best to catch these signs as early as possible. **Use the space below to identify what anxiety looks like for you:**

What do you notice yourself doing or *not* doing when feeling anxious? _____
_____
What physical symptoms do you experience? _____
What thoughts might you have? _____
What events seem to trigger anxiety? _____

Now that you've recognized when you're feeling anxious, there are several strategies you can use to reduce physical distress, overwhelm, and avoidance.

Coping Strategies: Activities you can *do* to reduce anxiety over the short and long term.

1. **Reduce physical distress** (e.g., mindfulness): _____
2. **Reduce overwhelm** (e.g., set small goals): _____
3. **Reduce avoidance** (e.g., exposures): _____

Helpful People: Reach out to people you feel safe with for support when you're feeling overwhelmed.

1. Name and phone #: _____
2. Name and phone #: _____
3. Name and phone #: _____

Helpful Resources: Keep a list of important contacts for when you need extra support.

1. Therapist name and phone #: _____
2. Doctor's name and phone #: _____
3. College Counseling Center phone #: _____

Coping With Anxiety as a Parent

As the parent of a child beginning college, you are likely to expect more independence from them while communicating with them less often. For many parents, this causes a significant uptick in worries related to their child's health, academics, and safety. Anxiety becomes problematic when anxious thoughts, feelings, and behaviors occur most of the day, nearly every day, and negatively impact your life. Symptoms to look out for include:

Anxious thoughts
(e.g., fear of your child being hurt, fear of failing as a parent)

Physical symptoms
(e.g., headaches, stomach aches, restlessness, quicker breathing/heartbeat)

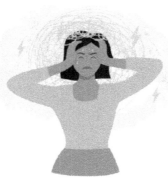

Difficulty concentrating

Avoidance behaviors
(e.g., delaying visits to campus, avoiding clear boundaries with child, refraining from providing your child with independence)

Identifying the signs of anxiety is crucial to seeking the right support, and it's best to catch these signs as early as possible. Use the space below to identify what anxiety looks like for you:

What do you notice yourself doing or *not* doing when feeling anxious? _____
_____
What physical symptoms do you experience? _____
What thoughts might you have? _____
What events seem to trigger anxiety? _____

Now that you've recognized when you're feeling anxious, there are several strategies you can use to reduce physical distress, overwhelm, and avoidance.

Coping Strategies: Activities you can *do* to reduce anxiety over the short and long term.

1. **Reduce physical distress** (e.g., mindfulness): _____
2. **Reduce overwhelm** (e.g., set small goals): _____
3. **Reduce avoidance** (e.g., exposures): _____

Helpful People: Reach out to people you feel safe with for support when you're feeling overwhelmed.

1. Name and phone #: _____
2. Name and phone #: _____
3. Name and phone #: _____

Helpful Resources: Keep a list of important contacts for when you need extra support.

1. Therapist name and phone #: _____
2. Doctor's name and phone #: _____

The Importance of a Good Night's Sleep

Chapter Overview

- Sleep Difficulties
- Sleep Difficulties and ADHD
- Tips and Tricks to Improving Sleep
- Post-Chapter Activities

This chapter will focus on a few of the common sleep difficulties experienced by both adolescents and adults (i.e., insomnia, hypersomnia). Following a brief overview, there will be information about how ADHD impacts sleep and why college students with ADHD might be especially impacted by sleep disturbances. The chapter ends with recommendations for how students can prevent and address difficulties with sleep.

SLEEP DIFFICULTIES

There are various types of sleep difficulties that college students can encounter. These difficulties may be characterized by too little sleep, too much sleep, or disrutptions in a typical sleep-wake cycle.

Insomnia

One of the most common sleep conditions is insomnia. Insomnia is diagnosed when someone has difficulty falling asleep (i.e., for at least 20–30 minutes), difficulty staying asleep (i.e., waking up in the middle of the night and difficulty falling back asleep), or early-morning wakefulness (i.e., waking up too early in the morning without being able to fall back asleep). However, the mere presence of these difficulties is not enough to warrant a diagnosis. These symptoms must impact an individual's day-to-day life (e.g., impacting work or school performance, daily responsibilities, or interpersonal relationships). Additionally, these sleep difficulties must be present for at least three days a week for three months. Short-term or occasional insomnia is somewhat normative; when someone is experiencing an increase in stress at work or interpersonal conflicts it may temporarily impact their sleep. If it becomes a chronic and impairing issue, then it may warrant working with a professional.

Hypersomnia

Hypersomnia is on the opposite end of the sleep difficulty spectrum. Rather than experiencing difficulties from too little sleep, an individual has trouble with excessive sleepiness even though they are getting a typical night's sleep. Specifically, for an individual to be diagnosed they need to experience one of the following despite sleeping 7 hours the night before: (1) taking naps throughout the day, (2) sleeping more than 9 hours but not feeling refreshed, or (3) difficulty being fully awake throughout the day. Being sleepy and needing more sleep is also normative at times, especially after a previously busy week or staying up late to study. To be diagnosed, these symptoms must be occurring three days a week for at least three months and impact an individual's day-to-day functioning (e.g., work, school, relationships).

Circadian Rhythm Disorders

Circadian rhythm difficulties are characterized by problems with one's internal clock and having a sleep-wake cycle that interferes with their daily life. One's sleep-wake cycle is impacted by their environment (e.g., when the sun rises or sets) or routines (e.g., when one eats, exercises, goes to work or school). In some cases, especially in college, students adopt a sleep-wake schedule that is not conducive to their academic or work-life. For example, a student might stay up until the early hours of the morning completing homework, playing video games, or watching TV or videos. Consequently, they are unable to get up in the morning for class and end up sleeping until late morning or even into the afternoon. As a result, they may miss classes or other obligations that take place earlier in the day. This becomes especially problematic if this off schedule becomes a habit (i.e., they repeat this schedule to the point that it becomes routine). Subsequently, it may become difficult for students to go to bed at a reasonable hour even if they attempt to do so. If students wake up late in the day (e.g., midafternoon), they may not feel physically tired at 11:00 p.m. Circadian rhythm disorder is diagnosed when these difficulties are consistently occurring and lead to either excessive sleepiness or insomnia, and impairment in day-to-day functioning.

Subclinical Difficulties

The above sections outlined the diagnostic criteria for various sleep disorders. However, many teens will experience sleep difficulties that do not rise to the level of a diagnosable disorder. Though rates of diagnosed sleep disorders are roughly 10%, research has shown that 62% of college students report experiencing poor sleep (e.g., trouble falling asleep, not getting enough sleep). Sleep problems often lead to mental health problems and poor academic performance. This suggests that even if these sleep problems are not rising to the level of a diagnosis, they should still be addressed.

SLEEP DIFFICULTIES AND ADHD

As previously mentioned, a majority of college students experience some level of sleep difficulties. Research also suggests that college students with ADHD experience sleep problems at an even higher rate than their peers. This is likely due to a bidirectional relationship between ADHD and sleep difficulties: ADHD leads to difficulties with sleep, and difficulties with sleep exacerbate ADHD symptoms and related difficulties.

ADHD and Mental Health Affecting Sleep

There are several ways that ADHD hinders good sleep. First, if teens take prescription stimulants to treat their symptoms of ADHD, it's important to monitor when they are taking their medication. Taking their prescription too late in the day (or taking a booster dose in the evening hours) could make it difficult for teens to physically fall asleep at a reasonable time. Therefore, it's important for teens to take their medication early enough in the day to not affect their sleep.

In addition to the effect of stimulant medication, the downstream effects of ADHD symptoms can also disrupt sleep. For example, if students procrastinate completing an assignment throughout the day (or throughout the week) they may be forced to complete it the night before it's due, causing them to get to bed later than desired and not getting enough sleep. Similarly, if students do not plan out their assignments in an effective manner (i.e., they plan to complete work late into the evening), this could impact their ability to get a full night's sleep.

Lack of having a bedtime routine can also affect your teen's sleep. Many times, teens get sidetracked when getting ready for bed. They may lose track of time, begin scrolling on social media, or text a friend. They then realize hours later that they still haven't showered, brushed their teeth, or started their bedtime routine. The opposite can also be true in the morning, in that students may opt to try and maximize their sleep as much as possible and not plan for the things they need to do to arrive at class on time.

Anxiety and depression that are sometimes secondary to ADHD symptoms may also affect sleep. Feeling anxious about the amount of work needing to get done or feeling depressed due to academic or interpersonal difficulties are feelings that are unfortunately not uncommon to untreated ADHD (see Chapters 14 and 15). The opposite can also be true here too. Sleep disturbances are symptoms of anxiety and depression, and may lead to either too much or too little sleep. These symptoms may lead teens to not want to get out of bed and not have the motivation to go to class and complete work, or make it difficult for them to fall asleep.

Sleep Affecting ADHD and Mental Health

Not only may ADHD impact sleep; sleep difficulties may also impact symptoms of ADHD. One of the hallmark traits of ADHD is difficulty paying attention. Sleep undoubtedly affects concentration. Lack of sleep can make these troubles with attention even more pronounced. This can make listening, engaging, taking notes in class, and completing assignments even more difficult.

Sleep also affects symptoms of depression and anxiety. When one is tired, it becomes more challenging to regulate emotions. Being tired on top of being anxious or stressed makes one feel even more stressed or anxious. Being tired or sleepy may decrease one's motivation and cause them to withdraw further (see "Reverse the Spiral" figure in Chapter 14).

TIPS AND TRICKS TO IMPROVING SLEEP

Given the pivotal role that sleep plays in ADHD symptoms and related difficulties, it's important to address sleep concerns as they arise. As has been stated with other clinical concerns, if your teen's sleep difficulties are severe, they should be treated by a specialist. It is recommended that you consult with your teen's pediatrician, primary care provider, or mental health provider to ensure that they are receiving appropriate care. However, if your teen is experiencing occasional or mild sleep problems, the following tips may be helpful to steer your teen back to a good night's sleep.

Plan Ahead

It's recommended that you circle back to Chapters 6 and 7. Managing time more effectively and maximizing productivity will allow your teen to have more flexibility with their time in the evening. Accomplishing tasks in a timely matter could help to eliminate any competing demands when it is time to sleep. Work with a professional on developing these skills, if necessary, may also have downstream impacts on sleep.

In crafting their schedule for completing homework, it is important to work backward. For instance, if your teen wants to get eight hours of sleep and needs to be to class by 9:00 a.m., then your teen should be asleep by midnight so that they wake up at 8:00 to get ready, eat, and make it to their classroom. However, if it typically takes your teen 15 minutes to fall asleep, then they should be in bed by 11:45. If they need to shower and brush their teeth and get their backpack in order for the following day before bed and that takes 30 minutes, they should plan to get ready for bed at 11:15. It might be helpful to have alarms or reminders set on their phone at 11:00 and 11:15 reminding them they need to start getting ready for bed. It may also be helpful to plan to end their homework time early enough in the evening to have time to relax (e.g., texting friends, watching a show, going on social media) before needing to get ready for bed. The phone alarms and reminders will also help your teen not overindulge with the relaxation and prompt them when it's time to begin getting ready for bed.

Create the Right Environment for Sleep

As was discussed in Chapters 6 and 7 regarding studying and completing assignments, it's equally important to create the right environment for sleeping. First, it's recommended that teens keep all electronics off when it's time to sleep. Televisions, computers, and phones all serve as distractions. There is also some research to suggest that the blue light from electronics reduces sleepiness. Keeping these electronics away from bed may reduce the temptation to use them—and it will force teens to get up and out of bed to turn the alarm off in the morning. This can be helpful in preventing your teen from snoozing alarms too frequently, oversleeping, or accidentally turning off an alarm and subsequently missing or being late for class (or other obligations).

In general, teens should only use their bed for sleeping. It's important that teens find a workspace other than their bed to complete assignments and study (see Chapter 6). Bed should be thought of as the place for ultimate relaxation. By doing school-related tasks in bed, bed becomes a trigger for your teen's brain to be in work mode rather than in sleep mode. Making sure that there is a designated workspace helps to lessen this concern.

Stick to a Consistent Sleep Routine

Sleep problems are most easily avoided when teens have a consistent sleep schedule (i.e., going to bed and waking up at the same time every day). This is true even on the weekend; teens should try to get up within an hour or two of their typical weekday wake time. This consistency will help to ensure that their sleep cycles do not become negatively affected. It's also important that teens try to avoid naps. A nap during the day could cause teens to not feel tired at their usual bedtime and subsequently alter their routine. If they are tired, encourage your teen to power through the day and if necessary, go to bed an hour or so earlier as opposed to taking a nap in the middle of the day.

There may be times when your teen's sleep schedule gets interrupted—travel, a busy work week, and being sick could all cause your teen's routine to be disrupted. This is normal! However, encouraging them to get back into their routine is important. There also may be times that teens go to bed but are unable to fall asleep. It's recommended that if your teen isn't able to fall asleep within 30 minutes, your teen should get out of bed. While out of bed your teen should read a book, meditate, or do something relaxing. When they begin to feel tired, they should go back to bed. What your teen should avoid is tossing and turning in bed for hours and becoming frustrated if they can't fall asleep.

Address Anxiety and Deal with Depression

Refreshing your teen's memory about their coping plans with anxiety and depression may also help to alleviate difficulties with falling asleep (or sleeping too much). In returning to the post-chapter activities for Chapters 14 and 15, you and your teen should discuss ways to alleviate stress or boost their mood. Addressing these mental health concerns could in turn improve their sleep. If their coping plans don't seem to be helping with their mood or their sleep, it may be time for you to help your teen seek help from a mental health professional for their anxiety or mood.

POST-CHAPTER ACTIVITIES

To prepare your teen to practice good sleep habits, review the "Sleep Quality Fact Sheet" with them. This worksheet will guide you through common sleep difficulties and offer tips for helping your teen establish a sleep routine. This content may need to be revisited once your teen begins college or if you notice poor sleep habits forming.

Remember to mark off the completion of this chapter and the corresponding worksheets on the "Preparing for College Checklist" (see Chapter 1). Be sure to have your teen save a picture of the completed worksheets in the designated spot on their phone or computer.

Sleep Quality Fact Sheet zZᶻz

A good night's sleep is essential for overall well-being and optimal functioning, especially for college students with ADHD. Quality sleep helps with focus, memory retention, and emotional regulation. This worksheet will provide you with a brief overview of sleep disorders to watch out for and tips to improve your sleep.

> **Common Sleep Disorders**
> - **Insomnia**: Difficulty falling asleep, staying asleep, or waking up too early that negatively affects daily life. It occurs at least three times a week for three months.
> - **Hypersomnia**: Excessive sleepiness despite adequate night sleep, characterized by frequent naps, sleeping over 9 hours without feeling refreshed, or difficulty staying awake. It occurs at least three times a week for three months.
> - **Circadian rhythm disorders**: Disruption of the internal clock leading to inconsistent sleep-wake cycles that interfere with daily activities.

Tips for Improving Sleep

- **Address anxiety and stress**
    - Practice relaxation techniques such as deep breathing, meditation, or progressive muscle relaxation.
    - Establish a consistent pre-sleep routine to signal to your body that it's time to wind down.
    - Plan for and complete assignments during the day rather than at night to avoid last-minute stress that can interfere with sleep.
- **End work early**
    - Set a specific time to stop working each evening to allow for wind-down time before bed. Use this time to engage in relaxing activities like reading, listening to music, or gentle stretching.
- **Manage time efficiently**
    - Prioritize tasks and create a schedule to balance academic responsibilities with relaxation. For tips on time management, refer to Part II of this book.
- **Avoid your phone and other electronics in bed**
    - Charge your phone away from your bed to avoid using it before sleep.
    - Use an alarm clock instead of your phone to wake up in the morning.
    - Do not do work, watch TV, or play on your phone while in bed to maintain a strong association between your bed and sleep.
- **If you can't fall asleep, get out of bed**
    - If you can't fall asleep within 30 minutes, get up and do a relaxing activity until you feel sleepy.
- **Get 7–8 hours of sleep**
    - Determine your wake-up time and plan backward to ensure a consistent bedtime and 7–8 hours of sleep (e.g., if your bedtime is 11:45 p.m., stop working at 10:00 p.m.).

- **Follow a consistent schedule**
    - o Go to bed and wake up at the same time every day, even on weekends, to regulate your internal clock.
    - o Set an alarm to begin your bedtime routine at the same time each night.
- **Avoid naps**
    - o Limit daytime naps to maintain your sleep schedule. If necessary, keep naps short (20–30 minutes) and early in the afternoon.

Alcohol Use

Chapter Overview

- How Does Alcohol Intoxication Occur?
- What Influences Levels of Intoxication?
- Alcohol and ADHD
- Deciding on Your Approach
- Post-Chapter Activities

With less parental or adult monitoring and easier access, college is a time when some students begin experimenting with alcohol. Though this may not be the case for all students, it's nonetheless important to talk about how alcohol may affect students (especially those with ADHD) and if they do engage in alcohol use, how they should do so safely. This chapter will provide the facts about alcohol use and suggestions for how to approach alcohol-related topics with your teen.

HOW DOES ALCOHOL INTOXICATION OCCUR?

To learn how to use alcohol safely, it is important to understand how alcohol intoxication occurs and what factors affect intoxication. Being intoxicated may result in bodily changes (physiologically, mentally, psychologically) that are in response to one's rising blood alcohol content (BAC). As one's BAC rises, their level of intoxication increases, so do the physiological, mental, and psychological symptoms. Our bodies have the ability to break down alcohol, but once there is too much alcohol in the bloodstream, the body cannot break it down quickly enough and you experience intoxication. The level of one's BAC is impacted by a variety of reasons, outlined in the next section.

WHAT INFLUENCES LEVELS OF INTOXICATION?

There are several factors that impact one's BAC or level of intoxication. The first may seem obvious: the number of drinks consumed. The more someone drinks, the more intoxicated (or drunk) they become. Though this is true, there are also many other (more nuanced) factors that impact intoxication.

Timing is an important consideration. Specifically, this refers to how one spaces their drinks out throughout an evening. Drinking one drink per hour helps students maintain a level of BAC below the legal limit for driving. However, there are even caveats to that; this is a rough guideline. Keeping your BAC in a moderate range generally means that it is okay for females to have 1 drink per hour for 3 hours; for males, this averages 1 drink per hour for 4 hours. After that time period and amount consumed, the body cannot keep up with breaking down the alcohol and BAC begins to rise much more rapidly. We won't get too complex here, but this is likely due to the fact that females have less of the chemical compound that breaks down alcohol than males do. Therefore, it's helpful for teens to try and stick to 1 drink per hour for 4–5 hours to remain at a moderate BAC level.

There are a few other factors that influence level of intoxication. The proof (or strength) of the alcohol increases the level of intoxication. An individual's BAC will rise slower when drinking alcohol of a lower proof compared to alcohol higher in proof. Body mass also influences one's BAC; individuals who have greater body mass may have slower increases in BAC. Consuming food prior to drinking alcohol is protective, because if there is food in one's stomach, that prevents BAC from rising more quickly.

ALCOHOL AND ADHD

Research has shown that among college students, those who have ADHD do not necessarily drink more alcohol than their peers without ADHD. However, those with ADHD are more likely to experience negative consequences related to alcohol use (e.g., missing class, not fulfilling obligations, doing or saying things they regret while under the influence of alcohol). The higher levels of alcohol-related negative consequences could be due to a variety of factors, many of which tie back to executive functioning (see Chapter 3). Research has suggested that disinhibition is one explanation. Disinhibition refers to one's level of impulsivity or ability to control their behavior. Compared to their peers without ADHD, college students with ADHD may act more impulsively or have more difficulty stopping drinking once they start. Difficulties in decision-making may also be a factor at play in the context of alcohol use and ADHD. This could be tied to differences in reward processing in individuals with ADHD. Research has suggested that because of differences in reward systems in the brain, students with ADHD may opt for a more immediate, short-term reward (e.g., having a fun night out drinking, watching television) over a more delayed, long-term reward (e.g., doing well on a test the coming week, getting a good grade on an assignment, passing a class).

DECIDING ON YOUR APPROACH

There are two different approaches to consider when talking with your teen about alcohol use during college: a "zero-tolerance" or a "protective behavioral strategy" approach. The decision is up to you as a parent. The following sections will outline the components of each approach and what the research says is most effective given your teen's current level of alcohol use. The zero-tolerance approach tends to be more effective for teens transitioning to college if they are engaging in only light or occasional alcohol use, or have not yet consumed any alcohol.

The alternative—introducing teens to protective behavioral strategies—tends to be more effective if they have already begun regularly experimenting with alcohol. With protective behavioral strategies, the implicit message is that you understand your teen is likely going to engage in alcohol use (i.e., you're not taking a zero-tolerance approach) and that they should learn methods to drink in the safest way possible.

You may choose to begin with a zero-tolerance discussion prior to your teen leaving for college. You may want to continue emphasizing that message throughout your teen's college years. However, you may eventually need to shift to a protective behavioral strategies approach if you learn that your teen is engaging in more frequent alcohol use. Your teen's thoughts or behaviors regarding alcohol use may shift throughout their time at college, and thus you need to be flexible in your approach over time.

Zero-Tolerance for Alcohol Use

A parental message of abstinence is one effective strategy for reducing the likelihood of your teen starting alcohol use or engaging in problematic alcohol use. These messages consist of parents expressing their zero-tolerance policy for alcohol use (e.g., "you should be refraining from alcohol use entirely while you are underage"). These messages seem to be most effective when delivered by parents to teens who have not yet initiated any alcohol use or who engage in only light drinking.

In addition to conveying these messages, it may be helpful for your teen to have some knowledge of learning refusal skills. These skills refer to ways in which teens should respond when offered (or pressured) to engage in alcohol use. Responses can be truthful in nature (e.g., "I don't drink," "I don't feel like drinking tonight," "Alcohol just doesn't do it for me, no thanks"). However, sometimes teens have difficulty providing these sorts of genuine answers. Teens may find it easier to come up with a fake excuse as to why they can't be drinking (e.g., "I have to be up early for class tomorrow," "I need to study all day and can't be hungover"). Either way, having a few canned responses may be helpful for when peers are pressuring them to drink.

It may also be helpful for your teen to purposefully plan activities that don't involve alcohol use, or to make friends with peers that do not engage in alcohol. Too often, students become trapped in a cycle where they are only attending events or parties that involve drinking. It is important that students try and schedule alcohol-free activities during their week to avoid falling into this trap. Having an inventory of activities may help ensure that your teen has options for spending their free time that don't involve drinking. It may also be helpful to schedule these activities with peers who have similar values around alcohol use. Cultivating a group of friends who do not use alcohol will make it easier for your teen to abstain.

Protective Behavioral Strategies for Alcohol Use

Strategies for reducing risky or problematic alcohol use are often referred to as protective behavioral strategies. These strategies are designed to decrease the severity or likelihood of negative consequences in response to alcohol consumption. In other words, they are guidelines or tips that students should follow to use alcohol as safely as possible. In some cases, introducing these strategies may be more effective than adopting a zero-tolerance policy for alcohol use. This has been shown to be the case when teens are already engaging in regular alcohol use. The idea of introducing protective behavioral strategies isn't indicative that you are encouraging your teen to use alcohol. Rather, it's providing teens with the knowledge of how to use these substances safely.

Teens may want to consider using a variety of the following strategies to reduce the risk of negative consequences related to alcohol use. The first and perhaps most obvious strategy is to set a personal limit as to the number of drinks your teen plans to consume. For example, your teen may want to commit to only drinking three or four drinks on a night out or at a party. They could do this by keeping a mental log or bringing a set number of drinks with them.

Knowing what is in a drink is important—and it's important that teens not accept drinks from people they don't know. These drinks may contain other substances that could be harmful to your teen. They might also contain an amount of alcohol that they are not expecting (i.e., the drink might be much stronger or higher in alcohol content than your teen expects). Teens may want to avoid large batch drinks at parties (e.g., punch bowls) for the same reason. It's impossible for them to know what ingredients (and in what quantity) are in them.

Another protective behavioral strategy that your teen could use to reduce negative consequences is spacing out the number of drinks throughout an evening. This may consist of alternating between alcohol and water (or another nonalcoholic beverage) to slow down the rate of drinking and to keep a rising BAC at bay. Avoiding drinking games where large amounts or quick consumption of alcohol are encouraged is also an effective protective behavioral strategy. Further, avoiding drinking alcohol straight (e.g., taking shots) can also space out alcohol consumption. Ensuring that food is consumed before drinking alcohol is also protective and reduces the risk of becoming intoxicated quickly. Your teen should avoid drinking on an empty stomach.

Consuming alcoholic beverages with high amounts of caffeine (e.g., mixing alcohol with energy drinks) or stimulant medication is dangerous, because they can mask the subjective feelings of intoxication and increase the risk for negative consequences related to alcohol use. In other words, high amounts of caffeine or stimulants lead an individual to feel more alert and less intoxicated than they actually are. In turn, this could lead to high levels of BAC, alcohol poisoning, and other harmful effects.

Teens should be mindful of their mood when they are engaging in alcohol use. For example, feeling unhappy, stressed, or depressed before drinking alcohol is associated with a higher quantity of alcoholic beverages consumed. Therefore, it may be wise for your teen to be aware of their mood going into a drinking session. If they are experiencing a negative mood, it could be a good idea for them to avoid drinking during that time (or to be extracognizant of the quantity they do drink).

It is also important to highlight methods for keeping teens safe while under the influence of alcohol. The first is to ensure that they have a ride home from events where alcohol is being consumed. This may be ensuring that there is a designated driver who has not been consuming alcohol, or using a ride-sharing app to safely get home when walking is not an option. When walking home while under the influence of alcohol, students should always be accompanied by a friend or roommate and avoid walking alone. It can also be helpful for your teen to share your location with friends or family members when drinking alcohol.

POST-CHAPTER ACTIVITIES

Your first task is to determine whether you would like to use a zero-tolerance or a protective behavioral strategies approach when discussing alcohol use with your teen. As was mentioned earlier in the chapter, your approach may change throughout your teen's college years, but based on the information provided in this chapter, you should decide how you want to initially broach this subject. Once you've decided on the approach you'd like to use, collaboratively review the "Alcohol Fact Sheet" with your teen, asking your

Alcohol Use

teen what they know about alcohol use and filling in the blanks with the information on that worksheet.

Finally, you should complete one of the alcohol use prevention worksheets: The "Alcohol Alternatives: Activities and Refusal Techniques" or "Using Alcohol Safely" worksheets. If you opt to choose the zero-tolerance approach, you should use the "Alcohol Alternatives: Activities and Refusal Techniques" worksheet and use language like, "As you transition to college, you may be confronted with situations where there is alcohol available. I hope that you use the following strategies to refrain from engaging in underage drinking." The worksheet provides discussion points for you and your teen and brainstorming ideas that can help prevent their alcohol use during college.

If you chose to adopt a protective behavioral strategies approach, "Using Alcohol Safely" should be used to facilitate discussion. If using this approach, you may want to use language like, "As you transition to college, you are likely going to be in situations where there is alcohol. I hope that you're open to talking about some ways for you to use alcohol as safely as possible." The corresponding "Protective Behavioral Strategy" worksheet outlines the protective behavioral strategies that you and your teen should discuss.

Remember to mark off the completion of this chapter and the corresponding worksheets on the "Preparing for College Checklist" (see Chapter 1). Be sure to have your teen save a picture of the completed worksheets in the designated spot on their phone or computer.

Alcohol Fact Sheet

While not everyone uses alcohol, it is often present in some social settings on college campuses. It's important to understand how alcohol affects your body so that you can make your safest and smartest choices. For students with ADHD, understanding these effects is crucial, as impulsivity and differences in reward processing can make managing alcohol use more challenging.

The amount of alcohol in your bloodstream is measured using **Blood Alcohol Content (BAC)**. As you consume alcohol your BAC rises, leading to various levels of intoxication. The factors depicted below can all influence your BAC:

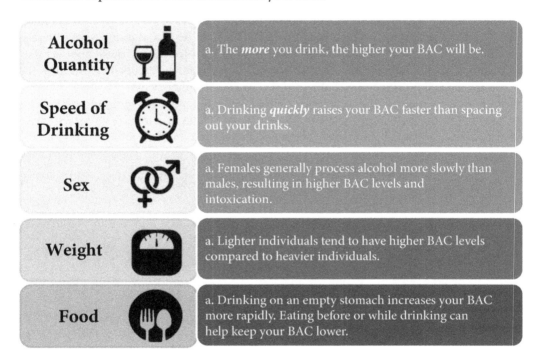

Drinking no more than one standard drink per hour (up to 3 for women or 4 for men) helps keep a person's BAC in a moderate range. The human body can't process more than one drink per hour; if you exceed this rate, your BAC will rise even faster. BACs under .05 are considered moderate. At this level, people report feeling relaxed and social, and although driving may be impaired, they feel generally in control of their actions. Once someone's BAC goes over .05, the more negative effects of alcohol become noticeable.

Note: Stimulant medications (and other medications) can affect how drunk you feel, even if your BAC remains the same.

Alcohol Alternatives: Activities and Refusal Techniques

As you transition to college, you may be confronted with situations where alcohol is available. Since we know that underage alcohol use can lead to negative health effects and academic issues, you can use some of the strategies on this worksheet to refrain from underage drinking. Use the spaces below to practice refusal skills and purposefully plan alcohol-free activities.

Refusal Skills

Refusal skills are essential tools that help you say no to underage drinking and make healthier choices. Here are some examples:

- "I don't drink."
- "I don't feel like drinking tonight."
- "I have to be up early for class tomorrow."
- "I need to study all day and can't be hungover."

Use the space below to write down your own refusal sentences. Writing them down can make it easier to remember and access in real-life situations.

1. _____
2. _____
3. _____
4. _____

Purposeful Activities

It can be easy to get swept up in a cycle of attending events with alcohol. Planning and participating in alcohol-free activities, particularly with peers who prefer not to drink, can lead to more meaningful college experiences. Here are some examples:

- Movie nights at the campus student center
- Intramural sports leagues
- Club meetings and social events
- Campus-sponsored concerts or performances

Use the space below to write down alcohol-free activities you might be interested in:

1. _____
2. _____
3. _____
4. _____

Using Alcohol Safely

As you transition to college, you are likely going to be in situations where alcohol is present. Therefore, it is important to talk about some ways for you to use alcohol as safely as possible. **Protective behavioral strategies** are actions you can take to minimize the risks and negative consequences associated with drinking alcohol. Review the list of strategies below and consider which ones may be most useful to you.

- **Count/Limit Drinks**
  Keep track of how many drinks you've had and set a limit for yourself before you start drinking.
- **Don't Drink Large Batch Drinks**
  Avoid punch bowls or communal drinks where you can't control the amount of alcohol.
- **Don't Accept Drinks from Strangers**
  Only take drinks from trusted friends or make your own to avoid unwanted substances.

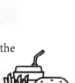

- **Space Drinks, Drink Water in Between**
  Alternate alcoholic drinks with water to stay hydrated and slow your alcohol consumption.

- **Avoid Shots**
  Shots can lead to rapid intoxication; stick to drinks you can sip slowly.
- **Avoid Drinking Alcohol with Highly Caffeinated Mixers**
  Mixing alcohol with energy drinks or other caffeinated beverages can mask the effects of alcohol, leading to overconsumption.
- **Eat Food Before Drinking**
  Having a meal before drinking helps slow the absorption of alcohol in your bloodstream.

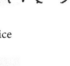

- **Be Mindful of Your Mood Before Beginning to Drink**
  If you're feeling down or stressed, consider whether drinking is the best choice for your emotional state.
- **Ensure a Ride Home (Designated Driver)**
  Plan ahead to have a safe way to get home, whether it's a designated driver, ride-share service, or public transportation.

- **Walk Home with a Friend**
  If you're walking home, make sure to do so with a friend for added safety.

PART VI

Ongoing Discussions

18

When and How to Revisit Content

Chapter Overview

- Revisiting Content
- Communication During College
- Post-Chapter Activities

If you've reached this chapter, you've covered the basics of helping your teen transition to college. Congratulations! I hope that you feel empowered and confident as your teen moves into their college years. To ensure your teen thrives, it may be important to regularly revisit these chapters throughout their time in school.

REVISITING CONTENT

It's hard to predict if and when you will need to review this content with your teen. Some chapters may need to be revisited frequently. For example, if you notice that communication with your teen is becoming strained, you may want to reexamine Chapter 2, which focuses on communication techniques. You and your teen may also want to reflect on their goals periodically (e.g., every semester) to tie their academic performance and social interactions back to what they hope to accomplish. You also may want to recall the class preferences discussed in Chapter 11 each semester as your teen is registering for courses.

It's likely that checking in on organization (Chapters 5 and 6) will be necessary when your teen begins college. Even if your teen practices these organization skills in high school, when their workload changes in college, they may need a refresh. As your teen approaches new types of assignments and tests, it may be helpful to review study, note-taking, and reading strategies (Chapter 7). If your teen is struggling with completing work on time or finishing tests and they were reluctant to register for accommodations, you could revisit the conversation about visiting the campus disability services office (Chapter 12). Similarly, it may be helpful to remind them of the resources on campus if you notice them struggling academically or socially (Chapters 10 and 12).

If your teen ultimately decides they want to be evaluated for stimulant medication or work with a professional on academics or other ADHD-related difficulties, you may want to revisit Chapter 13 on initiating mental health care. Likewise, if your teen begins to experience other mental health difficulties (e.g., depression, anxiety, sleep, alcohol), you and your teen could return to Chapters 14, 15, 16, or 17. Reminding them of their coping plans or sleep strategies could be helpful if you notice troubles in these areas. Checking in periodically on your teen's mental health will also normalize discussing these areas.

COMMUNICATION DURING COLLEGE

One of the most difficult aspects of the transition to college is balancing your teen's autonomy with wanting to monitor and support them. Your teen is likely looking for more independence and less supervision on their homework and class attendance. On the other hand, you may be concerned with your teen attending class and keeping up with schoolwork. You and your teen may be on opposite ends of the spectrum when it comes to level of parental involvement desired. Therefore, it would be helpful to discuss how often and how they want to be checked in on. Will they reach out to you with concerns, or will you send a daily text to see how homework is going? Negotiating a communication plan may help to reduce conflicts associated with this balance between independence and monitoring.

This communication plan may also need to change throughout college. Your teen may need more support in the beginning of their transition to college, with check-ins tapering off as they learn to manage their workload. For example, parents and teens might begin the college transition with daily check-ins with parents asking teens what work they need to accomplish and when they will complete it. As teens master completing their work on time, these check-ins may shift to a weekly basis. Similarly, parents may want to view their teen's college platform (i.e., Blackboard, Canvas) together each week to ensure that work is turned in on time and that there are no outstanding assignments. As work is being regularly completed and on time, parents may reduce this level of monitoring to once monthly (or eventually not requiring this monitoring at all). Parents and teens should arrive at the level of checking in and monitoring collaboratively and discuss how much tapering should occur and when (i.e., what benchmarks parents need to see to feel comfortable tapering off).

It's possible that you and your teen might discuss a communication plan that turns out to be ineffective, and it becomes evident that more monitoring is necessary. This could result from beginning at a place with too little communication or monitoring. It could also be the result of tapering off with check-ins too much or too quickly. Amping up the level of communication or monitoring should be completed collaboratively, with parents and teens arriving at a decision that is mutually agreed-upon. The post-chapter activity will guide you through this discussion.

Part of your communication plan should include how you and your teen will know when additional support is needed. You and your teen should be able to recognize the signs that things are going well as well as the signs that your teen is struggling. This discussion should encompass all areas of their life, including academics as well as their social life and general mental health.

POST-CHAPTER ACTIVITIES

As a final activity in this book, you and your teen should complete the "Communication Plan" worksheet where you and your teen should decide on how and when you will check in with your teen on their schoolwork and progress in college. You and your teen should discuss the signs that things are going well and the signs that your teen may need extra support for academics or mental health. This may include knowing when to reach out to a mental health professional for assistance.

Remember to mark off the completion of this chapter and the corresponding worksheets on the "Preparing for College Checklist" (see Chapter 1). Be sure to have your teen save a picture of the completed worksheets in the designated spot on their phone or computer.

Communication Plan

This communication contract can be used to outline mutually agreed-upon check-in schedules, preferred communication methods, and the signs to watch for that indicate college is or is not going well. The hope is that this contract helps you and your parent stay on the same page, allowing your parent to provide you with support when you need it.

1. **Check-In Frequency:**
   Decide on a regular check-in schedule (e.g., weekly, bi-weekly, monthly) to discuss academic progress and challenges.
   - Regular check-in time(s): _____

2. **Initiation of Check-Ins:**
   Determine who will initiate check-in conversations. Then, consider specific situations when the parent should initiate check-ins (e.g., after midterms, when grades are posted).
   - Who will initiate: _____
   - Specific situations for parent-initiated check-ins: _____
   _____

3. **Preferred Communication Method:**
   Agree on the preferred method of communication for check-ins to ensure clarity and comfort for both parties.
   - Text   - Phone call   - Video chat   - Other: _____

4. **Signs Things Are Going Well:**
   Identify indicators that signify academic and emotional well-being (e.g., consistently attending classes, meeting deadlines, expressing positive or neutral feelings about life).
   - _____
   - _____
   - _____

5. **Signs Things Are Not Going Well:**
   Identify warning signs that indicate potential struggles (e.g., frequently missing classes, a decline in grades, becoming withdrawn, expressing negative feelings about life).
   - _____
   - _____
   - _____

6. **When to Reach Out for Professional Help:**
   - ADHD-related concerns: _____
   - Other mental health concerns (e.g., anxiety, depression): _____
   _____

BIBLIOGRAPHY

American Psychiatric Association. (2022). *Diagnostic and statistical manual of mental disorders* (5th ed., text rev.). https://doi.org/10.1176/appi.books.9780890425787

American Psychiatric Association. (2024, April). *Find a psychiatrist.* https://finder.psychiatry.org/s/

American Psychiatric Association. (2024, April). *What is depression.* https://www.psychiatry.org/patients-families/depression/what-is-depression

American Psychological Association. (2024, May). *Psychologist locator.* https://locator.apa.org/

Anastopoulos, A. D., DuPaul, G. J., Weyandt, L. L., Morrissey-Kane, E., Sommer, J. L., Hennis Rhoads, L., Murphy, K. R., Gormley, M. J., & Gyda Gudmundsdottir, B. (2018). Rates and patterns of comorbidity among first-year college students with ADHD. *Journal of Clinical Child & Adolescent Psychology*, 47(2), 236–247. https://doi.org/10.1080/15374416.2015.1105137

Anastopoulos, A. M., Langberg, J. M., Besecker, L. H., & Eddy, L. D. (2020). *CBT for College students with ADHD: A clinical guide to ACCESS.* Springer.

Association for Behavioral and Cognitive Therapies. (2024, April). *Find a CBT therapist.* https://services.abct.org/i4a/memberDirectory/index.cfm?directory_id=3&pageID=3282

Bamber, M. D. & Morpeth, E. (2019). Effects of mindfulness meditation on college student anxiety: A meta-analysis. *Mindfulness*, 10, 203–214. https://doi.org/10.1007/s12671-018-0965-5

Becker, S. P., Jarrett, M. A., Luebbe, A. M., Garner, A. A., Burns, G. L., & Kofler, M. J. (2018). Sleep in a large, multi-university sample of college students: Sleep problem prevalence, sex differences, and mental health correlates. *Sleep Health*, 4(2), 174–181. https://doi.org/10.1016/j.sleh.2018.01.001

Benson, K., Flory, K., Humphreys, K. L., & Lee, S. S. (2015). Misuse of stimulant medication among college students: A comprehensive review and meta-analysis. *Clinical Child and Family Psychology Review*, 18, 50–76. https://doi.org/10.1007/s10567-014-0177-z

Bodalski, E. A., Flory, K., & Meinzer, M. C. (2023). A scoping review of factors associated with emotional dysregulation in adults with ADHD. *Journal of Attention Disorders*, 27(13), 1540–1558. https://doi.org/10.1177/10870547231187148

Canu, W., Knouse, L. E., Flory, K., & Hartung, C. M. (2023). *Thriving in college with ADHD: A cognitive-behavioral skills manual for therapists.* Routledge.

Children and Adults with ADHD. (2024, May). *Find an affiliate.* https://chadd.org/affiliate-locator/

Cuijpers, P., Muñoz, R. F., Clarke, G. N., & Lewinsohn, P. M. (2009). Psychoeducational treatment and prevention of depression: The "coping with depression" course thirty years later. *Clinical Psychological Review*, 29(5), 449–458. https://doi.org/10.1016/j.cpr.2009.04.005

DuPaul, G. J., Gormley, M. J., Anastopoulos, A. D., Weyandt, L. L., Labban, J., Jaffe Sass, A., Busch, C. Z., Franklin, M. K., Postler, K. B. (2021). Academic trajectories of college students with and without ADHD: Predictors of four-year outcomes. *Journal of Clinical Child & Adolescent Psychology*, 50(6), 828–843. https://doi.org/10.1080/15374416.2020.1867990

DuPaul, G. J., Gormley, M. J., & Laracy, S. D. (2013). Comorbidity of LD and ADHD: implications of DSM-5 for assessment and treatment. *Journal of Learning Disabilities, 46*(1), 43–51.

Gaultney, J. F. (2010). The prevalence of sleep disorders in college students: Impact on academic performance. *Journal of American College Health, 59*(2), 91–97. https://doi.org/10.1080/07448481.2010.483708

Gaultney, J. F. (2014). College students with ADHD at greater risk for sleep disorders. *Journal of Postsecondary Education and Disability, 27*(1), 5–18.

Jansen, D., Petry, K., Ceulemans, E., Van der Oord, S., Noens, I., & Baeyens, D. (2017). Functioning and participation problems of students with ADHD in higher education: which reasonable accommodations are effective? *European Journal of Special Needs Education, 32*(1), 35–53. https://doi.org/10.1080/08856257.2016.1254965

Johnston, C., Williamson, D., Noyes, A., Stewart, K., & Weiss, M. D. (2018). Parent and child ADHD symptoms in relation to parental attitudes and parenting: Testing the similar-fit hypothesis. *Journal of Clinical Child and Adolescent Psychology, 47*(S1), S127–S136. https://doi.org/10.1080/15374416.2016.1169538

Kim, J., Thompson, E. A., Walsh, E. M., & Schepp, K. G. (2015). Trajectories of parent-adolescent relationship quality among at-risk youth: Parental depression and adolescent developmental outcomes. *Archives of Psychiatric Nursing, 26*(6), 434–440. https://doi.org/10.1016/j.apnu.2015.07.001

Langberg, J. M., Dvorsky, M. R., Klipperman, K. L., Molitor, S. J., & Eddy, L. D. (2014). Alcohol use longitudinally predicts adjustment and impairment in college students with ADHD: The role of executive functions. *Psychology of Addictive Behaviors, 29*(2), 444–454. https://doi.org/10.1037/adb0000039

Li, S. T., Albert, A. B., & Dwelle, D. G. (2014). Parental and peer support as predictors of depression and self-esteem among college students. *Journal of College Student Development, 55*(2), 120–138. https://doi.org/10.1353/csd.2014.0015

Meier, S. M. & Deckert, J. (2019). Genetics of anxiety disorders. *Current Psychiatry Reports, 21*(16). https://doi.org/10.1007/s11920-019-1002-7

Miller, W. R. & Rollnick, S. (2012). *Motivational interviewing: Helping people change* (3rd ed.). Guilford Press.

Monk, R. L., Qureshi, A., & Heim, D. (2020). An examination of the extent to which mood and context are associated with real-time alcohol consumption. *Drug and Alcohol Dependence, 208*(1), 107880. https://doi.org/10.1016/j.drugalcdep.2020.107880

Morin, C. M. & Jarrin, D. C. (2022). Epidemiology of insomnia: Prevalence, course, risk factors, and public health burden. *Sleep Medicine Clinics, 17*(2), 173–191. https://doi.org/10.1016/j.jsmc.2022.03.003

Nagy, M. E. & Theiss, J. A. (2013). Applying the relational turbulence model to the empty nest transition: Sources of relationship change, relational uncertainty, and interference from partners. *Journal of Family Communication, 13*, 280–300. https://doi.org/10.1080/15267431.2013.823430

National Heart, Lung, and Blood Institute. (2024, May). *What are circadian rhythm disorders.* https://www.nhlbi.nih.gov/health/circadian-rhythm-disorders#:~:text=Circadian%%20rhythm20disorders%2C%20also%20known,cycles%20about%20every%2024%20hours.

National Institute of Mental Health. (2024, May). *Anxiety disorders.* https://www.nimh.nih.gov/health/topics/anxiety-disorders?rf=32471

Needham, B. L. (2008). Reciprocal relationships between symptoms of depression and parental support during the transition from adolescence to young adulthood. *Journal of Youth and Adolescence, 37*, 893–905. https://doi.org/10.1007/s10964-007-9181-7

O'Brien, M. C., McCoy, T. P., Rhodes, S. D., Wagoner, A., & Wolfson, M. (2008). Caffeinated cocktails: Energy drink consumption, high-risk drinking, and alcohol related consequences among college students. *Academic Emergence Medicine, 15*(5), 453–460. https://doi.org/10.1111/j.1553-2712.2008.00085.x

Pearson, M. R. (2013). Use of alcohol protective behavioral strategies among college students: A critical review. *Clinical Psychology Review, 33*(8), 1025–1040. https://doi.org/10.1016/j.cpr.2013.08.006

Phipps-Nelson, J., Redman, J. R., Schlangen, L. J. M., & Rajaratnma, S. M. W. (2009). Blue light exposure reduces objective measures of sleepiness during prolonged nighttime performance testing. *Chronobiology International, 26*(5), 891–912. https://doi.org/10.1080/07420520903044364

Psychology Today. (2024, May). *Find a therapist.* https://www.psychologytoday.com/us

PSYPACT. (2024, May). *PSYPACT Map.* https://psypact.org/mpage/psypactmap

Rooney, M., Chronis-Tuscano, A., & Yoon, Y. (2012). Substance use in college students with ADHD. *Journal of Attention Disorders, 16*(3), 221–234. https://doi.org/10.1177/1087054710392536

Safren, S. A., Sprich, S. E., Perlman, C. A., & Otto, M. W. (2017). *Mastering your adult ADHD: A cognitive-behavioral treatment program, therapist guide* (2nd ed.). Oxford University Press.

Shifrin, J. G., Proctor, B. E., Prevatt, F. F. (2010). Work performance differences between college students with and without ADHD. *Journal of Attention Disorders, 13*(5), 489–496. https://doi.org/10.1177/1087054709332376

Sieh, D. S., Visser-Meily, J. M. A., & Meijer, A. M. (2013). The relationship between parental depressive symptoms, family type, and adolescent functioning. *PLoS ONE, 8*(11), e80699. https://doi.org/10.1371/annotation/b8370232-c144-4c14-8168-8dceede5b8e2

Solanto, M. V. (2011). *Cognitive behavioral therapy for Adult ADHD: Targeting Executive dysfunction.* Guilford Press.

Tufty, L. M., Gallagher, V. T., Oddo, L., Vasko, J., Chronis-Tuscano, A., & Meinzer. M. (2024). Academic accommodations and functioning in college students with attention-deficit/hyperactivity disorder: Limitations, barriers, and suggestions for collaborators. *Journal of Postsecondary Education and Disability, 37*(1), 35–46.

Weyandt, L. L. & DuPaul, G. J. (2008). ADHD in college students: Developmental findings. *Developmental Disabilities Research Reviews, 14*, 311–319. https://doi.org/10.1002/ddrr.38

Wilens, T. E., Adler, L. A., Adams, J., Sgambati, S., Rotrosen, J., Sawtelle, R., Utzinger, L., & Fusillo, S. (2008). Misuse and diversion of stimulants prescribed for ADHD: A systematic review of the literature. *Journal of American Academy of Child and Adolescent Psychiatry, 47*(1), 21–31. https://doi.org/10.1097/chi.0b013e31815a56f1

Withers, M. C., Cooper, A., Rayburn, A.D., & McWey, L. M. (2016). Parent-adolescent relationship quality as a link in adolescent and maternal depression. *Child and Youth Services Research, 70*, 309–314. https://doi.org/10.1016/j.childyouth.2016.09.035

INDEX

Tables and boxes are indicated by an italic *t*, *f*, and *b* following the page/paragraph number.

academic accommodations
  access to, 112
  activities, 114
  barriers, 113–114
  distraction-reduced testing environment, 110
  excused absences, 111
  extended time on tests, 110
  flexible deadlines, 111
  helpful, 109–111
  how to use, 112–113
  note on learning disorders, 114
  note-taking resources, 110–111
academic coaching, 98
academic resources
  academic advising, 91
  disability resources center, 92
  office hours, 92
  tutoring and study sessions, 92
  writing assistance, 93
academics
  school selection, 69–70
  tasks list, 9*b*–10*b*
accommodations, 115. *See also* academic accommodations
accountability partners, task completion, 49–50
ACT (American College Testing), 82, 83
ADHD (attention-deficit/hyperactivity disorder), 3, 4, 5, 21
  activities, 25–26
  alcohol and, 152
  anxiety and, 136, 137, 140
  causes, 22
  college students with, 22–23
  depression and, 128
  description of, 21–22, 27
  example vignette, 24–25
  mental health and, affecting sleep, 146
  organizational system use, 37
  reading strategies for, 62, 64
  reflections on challenges and strengths, 28
  resources and support, 24
  sleep difficulties and, 145–146
  specialty services, 72–73
  strengths, 23, 28
  study strategies for, 62, 63
adulting, organizational system, 41–42
adult tasks, teaching basic, 4–5
advising
  academic, 91
  writing assistance, 93
alcohol fact sheet, 156
alcohol use
  activities, 154–155
  ADHD and, 152
  deciding on your approach, 152–154
  intoxication, 151
  levels of intoxication, 151–152
  protective behavioral strategies for, 152, 153–154
  purposeful activities, 157
  refusal skills, 157
  using alcohol safely, 158
  zero-tolerance for, 152, 153
American Psychiatric Association, 121
American Psychological Association, 121
Americans with Disabilities Act (ADA), 109, 115
anxiety. *See also* depression
  activities, 139
  ADHD and, 137
  addressing, 137–138
  coping with, 140–141
  coping with, as a parent, 142–143
  description of, 136
  parental, during the transition to college, 138–139

anxiety (*Continued*)
    sleep and, 148
application, tasks list, 9*b*
application checklist, 86
application forms, 81
appointments, organizational system, 40–41
Association for Behavioral and Cognitive Therapies, 121

blood alcohol content (BAC), 151, 156. *See also* alcohol use
    intoxication levels, 151–152
bullet journals, organizational system, 40

Calendar, 39, 40
campus resources. *See also* academic resources
    academic, 91–93
    activities, 96
    career services, 95
    community support, 94–95
    Information Technology (IT) office, 95
    logistical resources, 95–96
    mental health counseling, 94
    resident assistant, 95
    student health center, 93
career services, campus, 95, 99
Children and Adults with ADHD (CHADD) website, 121
circadian rhythm disorders, sleep, 145, 149
classes
    organizational system, 40–41
    practice making perfect, 61–62
    reading and re-reading, 61
    reading strategies for ADHD, 62, 64
    study strategies for ADHD, 62, 63
    taking notes, 60–61
class schedule
    activities, 102
    class schedule builder, 103, 104*t*, 105*t*, 106, 107*t*, 108*t*
    deciding on classes, 100–101
    selecting class times, 101–102
class size, college specialties for ADHD, 71–72
cognitive-behavioral therapy (CBT), 121, 124, 137
collaboration, 11
college(s). *See also* school selection
    communication during, 162
    term, 5
college application
    activities, 85
    application checklist, 86
    application forms, 81
    college essays, 82
    early decision and early acceptance options, 84
    letters of recommendation, 84
    necessities of, 85
    selected schools, 87, 88
    standardized tests, 82–84
college checklist, preparing for, 6, 8*b*–10*b*
college essays, college application, 82
college goals
    creating, 33–34
    weekly and daily, 34
college specialties
    class size, 71–72
    neurodevelopmental difficulties, 72–73
    school selection, 71–73
    specialty services for ADHD, 72–73
Common App, 81, 82, 84
communication
    activities, 162
    collaboration, 11
    decisional balance, 14
    during college, 162
    example vignettes, 15–17
    goals and, 12
    open-ended questions, 13
    positive approach, 13
    reflecting what you hear, 12–13
    revisiting content, 161
    rolling with resistance, 14–15
communication plan, 163
community support, campus, 94–95
conversation, reflecting what you hear, 12–13
coping
    anxiety, 140–141
    anxiety as a parent, 142–143
    depression, 132–133
    depression as a parent, 134–135
counseling center
    mental health, 94
COVID-19 pandemic, standardized tests, 82

daily responsibilities, organizational system, 41–42
decisional balance
    communication, 14
    practice quiz, 19, 20
decision-making tool, importance vs. urgency matrix, 55, 56

Index

depression. *See also* anxiety
  activities, 131
  addressing negative mood, 129
  addressing parental, 130
  ADHD and, 127, 128
  coping with, 132–133
  coping with, as a parent, 134–135
  description of, 127–128
  downward spiral, 129–130
  reversing the spiral, 129–130
  sleep and, 148
  upward spiral, 129–130
disability resource center, 92
  term, 109
distraction-reduced testing environment, 110
due dates, organizational system, 41

early action, college application, 84
early decision, college application, 84
electronic calendars, organizational system, 39–40
environment
  ideal for task completion, 48–50
  location, 48–49
  productivity factors, 50
essays, college application, 82
example vignettes
  ADHD discussion by parent and teen, 24–25
  communication, 15–17
  goal-setting, 30–32
  setting up organizational system, 43–44
exams, organizational system, 41
excused absences, accommodation, 111
extended time, accommodation, 110

fact sheet, alcohol, 156
Family Educational Rights and Privacy Act (FERPA), 139
finances, school selection, 71
flash cards, practice with, 61
flexible deadlines, accommodation, 111

goals, communication and, 12
goal-setting
  activities, 32
  creating college goals, 33–34
  example vignettes, 30–32
  types of goals, 29–30
  weekly and daily, 34
grade point average (GPA), 70
guidebook
  six parts of, 5–6
  topic areas, 3

homework, 101
  accountability partners, 49–50
  activities, 54
  breaking down tasks into manageable pieces, 52–53, 59
  creating the right environment, 48–50, 57
  importance vs. urgency matrix, 55, 56
  location, 48–49
  maximizing productivity, 53–54, 58
  prioritizing tasks, 50–52, 57, 58, 59
  productivity factors, 50
  rewards, 54, 59
  task completion skills for ADHD, 57–59
hypersomnia, 144–145, 149

Importance vs. Urgency Matrix, time management and decision-making tool, 55, 56
Individualized Education Plan (IEP), 109
Information Technology (IT) office, campus, 95
insomnia, 144, 149

learning disorders (LD), academic accommodations, 114
letters of recommendation, college application, 84
logistical resources. *See also* campus resources
  college, 95–96
long-term goals, 29, 30

medication use
  college, 122, 161
  diversion and safe storage, 123
mental health. *See also* depression
  ADHD and, affecting sleep, 146
  depression with ADHD, 127, 128
  tasks list, 9b
mental health care
  activities, 123
  initiating new care, 121–122
  medication diversion and safe storage, 123
  medication use during college, 122
  pharmacological care, 119–120, 126
  psychosocial therapeutic care, 120–121
  therapeutic care, 124
mental health counseling, campus, 94
mental health resources, 98
mid-term goals, 29, 30

mindfulness exercises, anxiety, 137
motivational interviewing, 5, 11

neurodevelopmental difficulties, specialty services, 72–73
Notes, 39
note-taking
    accommodation, 110–111
    classes, 60–61
    study strategy, 63

obligations, organizational system, 40–41
office hours, professors and teaching assistants, 92
Office of the Dean of Students, campus, 96, 99
open-ended questions, communication, 13
Organizational Skills Training (OST), 124
organizational systems
    activities, 45, 46–47
    bullet journals, 40
    classes, appointments and obligations, 40–41
    college students with ADHD, 37
    completing tasks, 41
    daily responsibilities (adulting), 41–42
    due dates and exams, 41
    electronic calendars, 39–40
    elements of, 40–42
    example vignette, 43–44
    initiating and maintaining, 42
    organizational skills discussion, 46–47
    paper calendars and planners, 39
    proactive completion, 42
    pros and cons of, 37–38
    sticky notes (Post-its), 40
    to-do lists, 39–40
    troubleshooting, 42–43
    types, 38–40

paper calendars, organizational system, 39
parental anxiety. *See also* anxiety
    coping with, 142–143
    during transition to college, 138–139
parental depression. *See also* depression
    addressing, 130
    coping with, 134–135
pharmacological care, maintaining, 119–120, 126
planners, organizational system, 39
positive reinforcement, task completion, 54
Post-its, organizational system, 40
practice, classes, 61–62

pre-college, tasks list for, 9*b*–10*b*
Premack principle, rewards, 54, 59
Preparing for College Checklist, 8*b*–10*b*
productivity
    factors, 50
    maximizing, 53–54
    task completion, 50
protective behavioral strategies, alcohol use, 152, 153–154
PsychologyToday, 121
psychosocial therapeutic care, maintaining, 120–121
PSYPACT organization, 120

reading, classes, 61
reading strategies for ADHD, 62, 64
Rehabilitation Act, Section 504, 109, 115
Reserve Officer Training Corps (ROTC), 71, 95
resident assistant, campus, 95, 99
resistance
    quiz on rolling with, 19, 20
    rolling with, 14–15
rewards, Premack principle, 54, 59
room and board, tasks list, 10*b*

SAT (Standardized Achievement Test), 82, 83
schedule. *See* class schedule
school selection
    academics, 69–70
    activities, 73
    application budget, 73, 74
    choosing a college, 73, 76
    class size, 71–72
    college budget, 73, 75
    college specialties, 71–73
    finances, 71
    general criteria for choosing, 69–71
    location, 70–71
    school data, 77*t*–80*t*
    specialty services for ADHD and neurodevelopmental difficulties, 72–73
Science, Technology, Engineering, and Math (STEM) classes, 101
short-term goals, 29, 30
sleep
    activities, 148
    ADHD and mental health affecting, 146
    affecting ADHD and mental health, 146
    anxiety and depression, 148
    creating the right environment for, 147
    planning ahead for, 147

Index

sticking to a consistent routine, 147–148
tips and tricks for improving, 146–148, 149–150
sleep difficulties. *See also* sleep
  ADHD and, 145–146
  circadian rhythm disorders, 145, 149
  hypersomnia, 144–145, 149
  insomnia, 144, 149
  subclinical difficulties, 145
sleep quality fact sheet, 148, 149–150
standardized tests, college application, 82–84
sticky notes, organizational system, 40
student health center, campus, 93
students
  note-taking, 60–61
  practicing problems, 61–62
  reading and re-reading, 61
study sessions, tutoring and, 92
study strategies for ADHD, 62, 63

task completion, 101. *See also* homework
  breaking into specific and manageable pieces, 52–53

combining importance and time-sensitivity, 51–52
importance, 51
organizational system, 41, 42
prioritization, 50–52
rewards, 54, 59
skills for ADHD, 57–59
time-sensitivity, 51
tasks list for pre-college, 9*b*–10*b*
terminology, writing style and, 5
timeline, suggested, for success, 7
time management, importance vs. urgency matrix, 55, 56
to-do lists, organizational system, 39–40
tutoring sessions, 92

universities. *See also* school selection
  term, 5

vocational schools, 5

writing assistance, 93
writing style, 5

zero-tolerance for alcohol use, 152, 153